A FIRST STEP

Understanding Guillain-Barré Syndrome

A fresh perspective on a devastating illness and eventual recovery… the triumph of Brian S. Langton.

A FIRST STEP

Understanding Guillain-Barré Syndrome

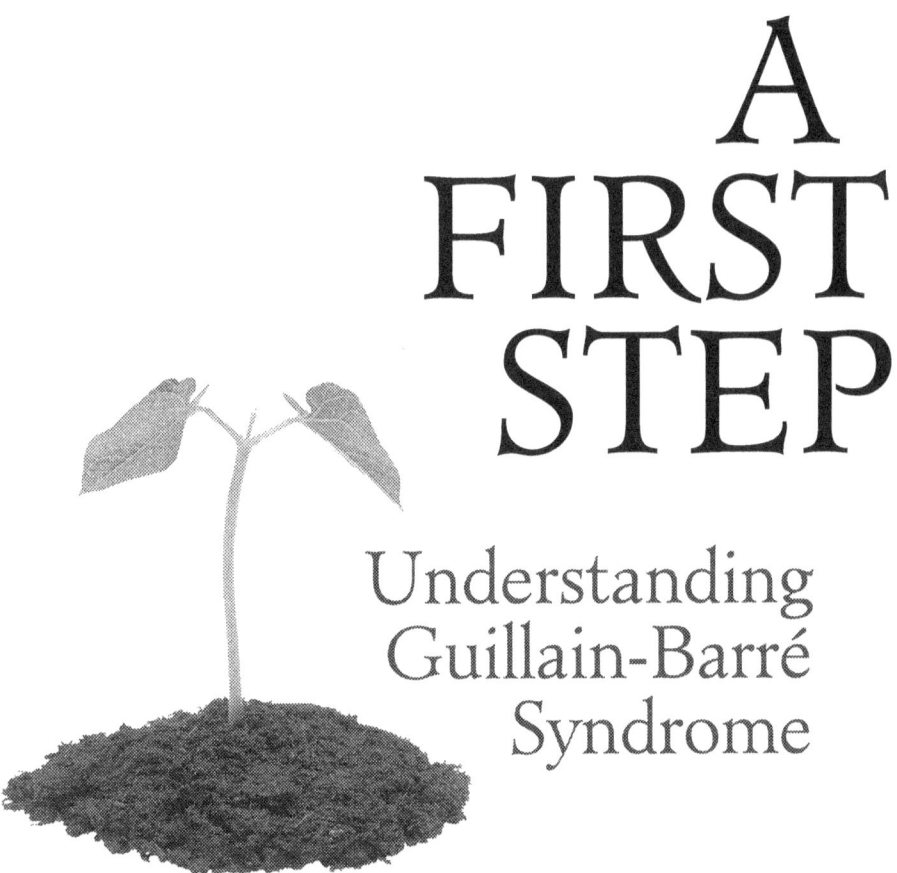

Brian S. Langton

A First Step: Understanding Guillain-Barré Syndrome
Author: Brian S. Langton

Copyright © 2002 Brian S. Langton. All rights reserved. No part of this publication may be reproduced, stored in a retrieval system, or transmitted, in any form or by any means, electronic, mechanical, photocopying, recording, or otherwise, without the written prior permission of the author, except by a reviewer, who may quote brief passages in a review. Contact the author in care of Trafford Publishing: Suite 6E, 2333 Government St., Victoria, B.C., Canada V8T 4P4.
Phone: 250-383-6864 • Toll-free: 1-888-232-4444 (Canada & US)
Fax: 250-383-6804 • E-mail: sales@trafford.com • Web site: www.trafford.com

Trafford Catalogue #02-0224 • Visit www.trafford.com/robots/02-0224.html to order.

This book was published on-demand in cooperation with Trafford Publishing. On-demand publishing is a unique process and service of making a book available for retail sale to the public taking advantage of on-demand manufacturing and Internet marketing. On-demand publishing includes promotions, retail sales, manufacturing, order fulfilment, accounting and collecting royalties on behalf of the author. TRAFFORD PUBLISHING IS A DIVISON OF TRAFFORD HOLDINGS LTD

Cover and interior design and production by Pneuma Books.
Set in Minister Light 11/14.

Disclaimer:
The Author is not a medical professional. All opinions expressed are his alone, unless specifically attributed to others. No liability will be accepted for persons acting in any manner whatsoever based on information contained in this publication.

* * *

National Library of Canada Cataloguing in Publication

Langton, Brian S., 1928-
　A first step : understanding Guillain-Barré syndrome / Brian S. Langton.

ISBN 1-55369-411-2

　1. Langton, Brian S., 1928- —Health. 2. Guillain-Barré syndrome—Patients—Biography. I. Title.

RC416.L35 2002　　　　　362.1'9687　　　　　C2002-902256-8

10　9　8　7　6　5　4　3

TRAFFORD

This book is dedicated to my wife, Sylvia, and our daughters Ruth, Kim, and Sally.

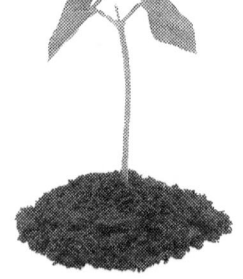

Table of Contents

* * *

Foreword xxi
Author's Preface xxxi

Part I — What Really Happened xxxiv
  1 A Rare Disease Hits 1
  2 What Is This Disorder? 9
  3 What Causes Guillain-Barré Syndrome? 15
  4 Destination: Intensive Care 21
  5 New Quarters 27
  6 As Bad As It Gets 37
  7 Patients, and Their Televisions 41
  8 The Art & Importance of Communicating 47
  9 Communication Journal Started 53
10 Humour Has Its Place 57
11 Learning to Talk Again 69
12 Encouragement from an Unexpected Source 81
13 Some Reflections on Life in Intensive Care 87
14 Approaching Yuletide 95
15 Better Days 109
16 Breathing on My Own 113
17 Light at the End of the Tunnel 117
18 Another Big Step Forward 123
19 GBS Patients are Neither Quadriplegics 127
      Nor Brain Damaged
20 A First Visit Home 133
21 Some Reflections on Life in the Rehabilitation Ward . 137
22 Was Guillain-Barré the Best Name for This Syndrome? 143
23 Changes Needed 149

24	The First Steps	153
25	Homecoming	157
26	Starting to Live Again	165
	Photographs	172

Part II — In Dreams 175
Introduction to Dream Sequences 177

27	GBS Patient on Secret Mission	181
28	Who Wants to Buy a Double-Decker Bus?	205
29	Submariner in Trouble	213
30	Guardian Angel in a Stetson	217
31	Sheriff's Office	223
32	Ottawa Summers	227
33	Quicksand Floor	233
34	Precious Stone	239
35	Underground Canal	245
36	Heavy Snowfall Warning	251
37	Downtown Adventures	259
38	Part Time Patient	267
39	Daylight Robbery	273
40	Neck Brace	279
41	Debt Collector	283
42	Flying Bombs	285
43	Across the Great Lake	289
44	A Game of Chicken	295
45	Jet Fighters On Call	299
46	Wild Dogs Attack	303
47	Catastrophe	311
	Photographs	318

Part III — Epilogue 321
Epilogue 323

Part IV — Appendices 327
Appendix 1: Endnotes 329

Appendix 2: Support Resources 337
Appendix 3: Internet Information Resources 353
Appendix 4: Reading List 365
Appendix 5: Guillain & Barré: The Namesakes 379
Appendix 6: Index 383
Appendix 7: About the Author 395

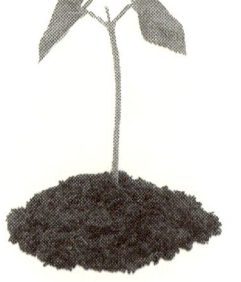

List of Photographs

∗ ∗ ∗

Photographs from Part I 172
   Outside with Physiotherapists and Caregivers 172
   Situated in the Car 172
   Outside With a Caregiver 172
   Two Occupational Therapists 173
   A Physiotherapist 173
   Outside with a Caregiver 173

Photographs from Part II 324
   F-16 on Runway 324
   Cockpit Check 324
   Taking Off 325
   View from Cockpit 325

∗ ∗ ∗

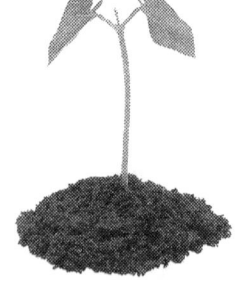

Acknowledgements

◆ ◆ ◆

"Friends are angels who lift us when our wings have forgotten how to fly." (Anonymous)

Grateful thanks to my family, especially my wife, Sylvia, who stood steadfastly by my side and throughout many emotionally charged days and months maintained the journal that has provided the basis for this book. We were an incredible team, working our way through a most unexpected life crisis. A big thank-you, also, to our friends and relatives who rallied to support Sylvia and me at a critical time.

I also want to acknowledge and thank the following:

> The doctors, nurses, and staff of the Intensive Care Unit at Foothills Hospital, Calgary, Alberta, Canada, for my early and accurate diagnosis and twelve days of thorough care and attention before being transferred to Rockyview;

> The doctors, nurses, and staff of the Intensive Care Unit at Rockyview General Hospital, Calgary, who for seven months provided phenomenal care and were part of my extended family. I thank them all, as well as the doctors, nurses, and staff of the rehabilitation team of Unit 58 at the Foothills Medical Centre, Cal-

gary, Alberta, who put up with me for almost four months as an in-patient;

Nancy, Elizabeth, Brenda, Julianne, Marlon, and so many others at Foothills for their encouragement and assistance;

Rosemary, my community physiotherapist, to whom I could always turn for advice.

Yi-nei and Kelly, who specialized in hand therapy at Rockyview General Hospital;

Emma and Katherine at the University of Calgary Rehabilitation and Fitness Program;

My dentist friend, Dr. Don Wallace, B.A., D.M.D., who not only took time out to visit, but also made 'house calls' to the hospital to provide needed professional care;

My business associates and colleagues for their giant-sized get well card containing over one hundred signatures and personal messages and for their concerns and assistance in so many very practical ways;

The players and staff of the then, and I hope soon to be again, English Premiere Division club, Nottingham Forest, for their good wishes and words of support;

My long-term caregivers, Cindy and Asunta for staying the course with their encouragement and caring support; and to Tara for her arm, which supported my first steps free of a walker;

··· Acknowledgments ···

Giselle LaBrie, for her care, encouragement and invaluable assistance in the planning and writing of this book at a time when 'my wings had forgotten how to fly';

Dr. Frank Warshawski MD, FRCPC, Director of Intensive Care, Rockyview General Hospital, Division of Respiratory Medicine and Department of Critical Care, Calgary Health Region, University of Calgary for his valuable support, advice, and encouragement and for his important contribution in writing the Doctor's Foreword;

Dr. Joel S. Steinberg, MD, PhD, Vice President and Director of the Guillain-Barré Syndrome Foundation International for his encouraging remarks and permission to reproduce excerpts from *GBS — An Overview for the Lay Person*, written by Dr. Steinberg and published by the Guillain-Barré Syndrome Foundation International;

Dr. Kopel Burk, MD, for his good advice and kind permission to reproduce excerpts from his paper "Communications and Altered Perceptions", originally published in the Journal of the Medical Society of New Jersey, *New Jersey Medicine*;

Luc Van Bavel, who kindly gave permission for the use of the F-16 and aerial photographs used in "G.B.S. Patient on a Secret Mission";

Anne Shard, RGN, for her encouragement and kind advice;

Margot, my chest physiotherapist in Intensive Care

at Rockyview Hospital, for her helpful advice and kind assistance;

Dr. J. B. Winer, MSc MD FRCP, Consultant Neurologist, University Hospital, Birmingham, England, for his kind permission to reproduce excerpts from his article, "The Early Years", which appeared in the Tenth Anniversary Issue of *Reaching Out*, April 1995, published by the G.B.S. Support Group of the U.K;

The Nottingham Evening Post, for their kind permission to reproduce excerpts from a feature originally published in November, 1998;

Andrea Robertson, RN, BN, for her valuable advice and encouragement;

Kim McLeod and Debbie Berge, Rockyview Hospital, Calgary;

Tara Butler, for her assistance with proofreading;

My editor, Jae Malone; and

Brian Taylor and the talented team at Pneuma Books.

I also wish to acknowledge all those friends, neighbours, or just concerned people, some of whom we hardly knew, who undertook acts of kindness in support of me and my family.

...

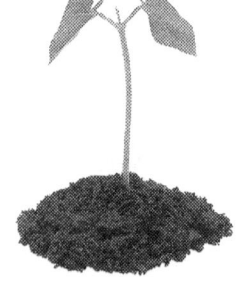

Foreword

* * *

This work by Brian is a true gift to humanity. Those who suffer this disease process have a unique experience, often very difficult and sometimes terrifying for themselves and their loved ones. To read this inside account is to have a chance to understand so much more, so much more quickly for patients, loved ones and caregivers alike. Yes, I certainly do not leave caregivers out amongst those who stand to benefit greatly from this clear and frank account. Guillain-Barré syndrome is not common and many medical personnel rarely if ever witness a case let alone act as a primary caregiver. Without experience or good reference sources we can all lose ground or suffer unneeded anxiety before expertise is obtained.

I first need to explain where I come from. I am an Intensive Care physician or now more commonly called a specialist in Critical Care. If you will, we are the general practitioners of the critically ill. We oversee all care coordinating the contributions of all the other disciplines of Medicine. We are responsible for anyone ill enough to require life support until they are stable enough to again be transferred to a bed on a hospital ward. Critical care specialists or 'Intensivists' come from a parent discipline such as Internal Medicine or one of its subspecialties including Neurology, Surgery, Anesthesia, Pediatrics or Emergency Medicine. We receive at least 2 extra years of specialized training and experience before assuming responsibility for critically ill patients. I trained in Internal Medicine including Neurology but subspecialized in Respiratory or Chest medicine before embarking on my career of patient care.

I explain the above to give you, the reader, a reference point from which to take my views.

To witness the struggle of Guillain-Barré, to truly involve oneself with it, is difficult for many physicians and other healthcare workers on several levels. On one hand you carry out daily visits to a patient who quickly slips into a state of apparent coma, unable to effectively communicate. Secondly, the daily work of care is carried out by many people — nurses, respiratory therapists, physiotherapists, social workers, spiritual advisors, ward aides and dieticians with communication and coordination being difficult to arrange. Finally change is seemingly glacial from day to day and new problems come up which can be extremely formidable.

To not overcome these hurdles is to miss the excitement of the disease, that of truly helping the unfortunate victim. To suddenly go from a healthy active lifestyle that you are working very hard to maintain with large expectations of great success, to helplessness in a matter of hours is frightening in the extreme. To many of the patients, going to prison would be easier and preferable, however these people have committed no crime.

Thus the focus early in the course is one of moral support whilst doing everything needed to rule out the other diagnoses of the differential, other conditions that can cause similar symptoms. Neurologists will spearhead this investigation with their strongest tools being the patient's history, examination and a test of the electricity of the muscles and nerves ('EMG' or electromyography and tests of the electrical conduction of nerves). Caregivers taking the time to speak at length to the patients and families trying to explain what has and will go on can be priceless at this stage.

The focus then clearly shifts quickly to a mode of care that many medical personnel in acute care areas do not cope well with — that of chronic care! Communication with the patient is difficult. Communication with the family and significant others is also often challenging. Family members often quickly become very stressed facing the conflicting goals of being at the hospital and carrying out the mandatory duties of their daily lives. Firm answers for most of their questions are hard to come by and most of the answers you do have are as difficult to hear as they are to deliver — 'We do not know what the exact cause is, cannot predict the course nor whether the treatments we offer, with their side effects, will help.'

For reference and reinforcement the reader needs a capsule summary of the medical facts of this entity. Guillain-Barré is an 'idiopathic' (meaning we do not know why), 'acute' (speaking to the abrupt onset of the disease not its course), 'inflammatory' (meaning it does its damage because of redness and swelling engendered by the body's own defense mechanisms including specialized cells like white cells and chemicals that the body makes and releases), 'demyelinating' (this is a tougher one — we in effect lose the biologic insulation from around our nerves in the body that carry signals out to tissues and back to the brain) 'polyneuropathy' (that is both motor and sensory nerves of different types are negatively affected). The brain itself is usually not affected, leaving the person, at first, entirely awake and aware but only variably able to sense their surroundings or react to them.

Guillain-Barré is characterized by progressive muscle weakness over hours to several days. Remission or improvement is really almost entirely 'spontaneous'; that is, the body heals itself — if given the opportunity. Seventy-five percent of patients do not get severe enough to need the Intensive Care Unit but multidisciplinary therapy is vital to ensure the best possible outcome.

Significantly, approximately two thirds of patients describe a recent respiratory (breathing) tract or abdominal infection.

Very importantly it must be stated that although Guillain-Barré has been reported to follow vaccination, specifically flu vaccination, this is not proven and has been overstated in the recent past. The most solid studies done to date show a possible (and I stress possible) increase in incidence of one per two million vaccinations. The number of cases of flu that are prevented, therefore preventing disability and death from that illness, far outweigh the risk and problems of Guillain-Barré. Every year flu vaccination programs are getting larger, however there is no apparent increase in the incidence of Guillain-Barré. It is therefore becoming ever more probable that even the extremely weak association between the two is incidental, not cause and effect.

The infection most commonly seen to precede Guillain-Barré is diarrhea with a bacteria of a family called 'Campylobacter'. Campylobacter bacteria are the leading cause of sudden diarrhea worldwide so it is difficult to avoid. It is a bacteria borne in food and carried in the bowels of a wide range of animals used for food all over the world.

If Guillain-Barré comes on in association with this bacteria it is also more likely that the patient may come down with the two most severe forms of the disease, that of 'axonal degeneration' and the 'Miller-Fisher' variant.

In the axonal form, that suffered by Brian, the insulation is lost off the nerves plus many of the nerve fibers themselves degenerate. This means in order to recover the nerve cell bodies in the spinal chord have to regenerate their nerve fibers before they can regenerate the insulation that covers them. Nerve fibers may not grow again or if they do, only very slowly, taking months to reform. In the time it takes this to happen changes such as muscle loss or contractors of limbs can be so severe that full function cannot be regained.

Miller and Fisher simply described cases of the disease that also affect directly some of the nerves of the brain. Some authorities believe the Miller-Fisher variant to possibly be a related but separate disease.

The deterioration of Guillain-Barré can vary in onset from hours to about two weeks; recovery is often within months but can stretch much longer. Besides weakness, difficulty with the nerves that control automatic body functions can lead to heart rhythm problems, difficulties with low or high blood pressure, unusual sweating, bowel function and bladder function and unusual sensitivity to some medications all of which must be managed carefully. These problems lead to a great deal of the problems (morbidity) and deaths (mortality) of this disease. A great deal of day to day difficulty can come from severe discomfort as nerves carrying sensory information (pain, light touch, pinprick, temperature and joint position) recover. Their messages can be somewhat scrambled leading to great discomfort. Brian at times suffered greatly with these 'dysesthesias'.

Critical illness and being on life support often affects the brain and one's perception of reality whether one suffers Guillain-Barré or the myriad of other problems that can lead to Intensive care unit admission. This brain dysfunction (or 'encephalopathy') of the critically ill is well known and characterized but not well understood. On a fundamental level it may be a defense mechanism of the psyche and represents the combined effect of anxiety, pain, sleep deprivation and the effects of drugs. Patients enter a state of altered perception of reality most often accompanied by amnesia. Brian's accounts of his reality during his illness are indeed remarkable.

Therapy with intravenous protein antibodies (gamma globulin) or washing antibody proteins out of the blood (plasmapheresis) is experimental and of low general effect and may be carried out depending on the nature and resources of individual hospitals.

About 15 percent of patients recover completely. Another 65 percent suffer minor deficits, which do not interfere significantly with quality of life. Five to ten percent are disabled and in spite of the best of care about six percent of patients die often in association with concurrent chronic illnesses or advanced age.

You can see that a focus of my recommendations for care follows the proven and recommended practice of taking whatever time is needed to communicate with patient and family. The downstream benefits are well worth the investment in time for all parties. The fact that the reader has picked up this book attests to the need and quest for information and I applaud your mission.

Another aspect of care, which has been very successful, is to, as early as possible once a firm diagnosis has been made, establish a well-coordinated and documented plan of weekly care. All services and family are involved in the process. Then, even when staff turns over, the greatest measure of consistency and thoroughness of care can be achieved. An erasable board is erected in the patient's room for all to see with a weekly schedule of times of various activities and goals.

As with all of patients, especially those of longer term, we entreat families to bring in photographs of the patient when they were well. This serves to help staff remember the patient's identity and humanity even when they are at their worst. We also mandate speaking in the patient's room always as though they were awake and cogent as, especially with this disease, you never know for sure when they are listening. Any discussions that, in your judgment, the patient should not hear are best held out of the immediate vicinity of the patient, in meeting rooms if necessary. This goes especially for medical staff that can sometimes wax lyrical without thinking of the impact of their discussion on partially informed ears that can take the words out of context. It can be confusing and at worst cause unnecessary anxiety on the part of the patient.

This information sharing and planning of care we hold always as a primary concern and we hold weekly or biweekly multidisciplinary meetings of staff and family to continue the process. If it appears the patient can cope and even participate these are held right in the patient's room. Honest and forthright answers can be heard by all at once, greatly increasing the clarity and consistency of communication. Even in the face of staff turnover and different people explaining the same thing differently, true communication and understanding can be accomplished.

The fostering of teamwork cannot be underrated. Resources are increasingly limited in health care as budgets fail to expand and cost increases. Innovation is the only relief if it can be mustered and a great team is a much more fertile ground for innovation than a disgruntled group of isolated individuals.

Research is carried out in many Intensive Care Units but should only be carried out with full consent and understanding of the patient (if possible) and family with the knowledge that failure to choose participation in research protocols in no way affects quality or quantity of care. The process must be open and informed and there must be no coercion. A standard to strive for in any worthy institution. Because of the nature of this disease with its cause still unknown, research has been vital in giving us the ability to help as much as we do and will of course be needed to truly some day treat or prevent it. For the benefit of patients yet to come I encourage all to consider participation with an open mind.

Brian had the axonal form of the disease. His survival, recovery, and the production of this work despite disability represents a mammoth effort of will.

The diaries kept by his wife are straight from the heart, a true representation of how the process was perceived from the inside. We all have these thoughts but many times they are lost before being documented. We are so thankful to know our feelings are shared which always to some extent relieves the burden.

Finally, as a physician twenty-five years into the practice of medicine I must acknowledge that one recovers well from this disease not so much from the hard work of knowledgeable caring physicians, but because of the day to day work of the whole team with non-physician members and the patient doing the vast lion's share of the work. The Critical Care environment is a great place to work simply because unsuited staff do not last. If you cannot do your job well and get along with others you quickly realize your talents are best suited elsewhere. We are left with a distillate of people who know and love their work and it is a privilege to be a part of it all.

I know this work can help relieve a burden for the reader, make life a bit easier and productive, and as always should be the aim of medical care, at least give some measure of comfort.

Frank J. Warshawski, MD, FRCPC
Director of Intensive Care
Rockyview General Hospital,
Division of Respiratory Medicine and Department Critical Care
Calgary Health Region, University of Calgary
August 2001

"I was never supposed to walk again, was I?"
"No you weren't, but then you don't listen, do you?"

— Conversation between the Author
and Physiotherapist, Brenda

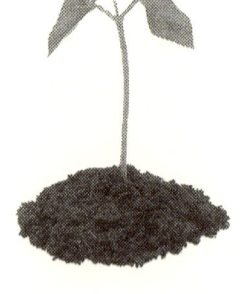

Author's Preface

After a few moments, the reader will quickly realize this is not a medical textbook. Having said that, I should also say that, being the frightening story of a rarely talked about disease told from the point of view of one who was suddenly stricken with almost total paralysis, it would not be out of place in the library of any medical professional.

While there is much technical information on the subject of Guillain-Barré Syndrome (G.B.S. for short) available in medical texts and journals, little has been written about the syndrome that explains, from a patient's perspective, what a sufferer, his family, and friends have to endure. My experience as such a patient shows me that not all nurses and therapists are familiar with G.B.S. and the unique needs of a patient afflicted with the syndrome. It is my hope that this publication makes a contribution towards filling that void.

Guillain-Barré patients, like me, who are unfortunate enough to experience the almost total paralysis that comes with one of the most severe forms — acute, chronic axonal G.B.S. — have unique needs. In addition to the inability to control body functions, they are unable to communicate. In my case, I could not speak, move my lips, my eyes or my arms. Writing messages, therefore, was out of question. I could not even wiggle my ears!

Thankfully the paralysis stopped short of affecting my brain. Fortunately, this is typical of the Guillain-Barré Syndrome.

I am convinced that having an active mind while virtually all body functions had shut down, caused me to experience a whole range of dreams, nightmares, and hallucinations, as though my brain had a compelling desire to stay occupied. These forays into 'alternate states' were so realistic that, in many cases, it was difficult, if not impos-

A First Step

sible, to distinguish them from reality. I have spoken to other patients with G.B.S., and they claim to have had similar experiences.

Some of the dream sequences — and I will use that phrase throughout this book, although many were actually nightmares — were hilarious, somewhat hilarious, or just plain scary.

This book is comprised of two distinct parts. Part I, 'What Really Happened', is a more-or-less blow-by-blow account of the effect Guillain-Barré Syndrome had on my close family and me from its surprise onset, through treatment and subsequent rehabilitation.

The second part of the book is devoted to describing some of those dream sequences referred to above. Because they take the reader into the mind of a G.B.S. patient, I believe they can provide further insights to medical professionals and interested readers about the inner experiences of long-term intensive care patients afflicted with Guillain-Barré Syndrome and other illnesses. Some of the needs and experiences of such patients may come as a surprise and contradict previously held beliefs. I'm certain that fellow G.B.S. sufferers and their families will relate to many of the situations described and have many similar stories of their own.

The decision to publish sprang from the need to encourage patients afflicted with this syndrome to face the future with optimism; to acknowledge the hard work necessary to get better; and, above all, to affirm the critical importance of a sense of humour. For those who accept the challenge, there is, indeed, light at the end of the tunnel. I firmly believe that with the right mindset, anything is possible.

Enjoy your read! Although the subject matter is serious, there is quite a lot of fun stuff between the covers.

The Author

...

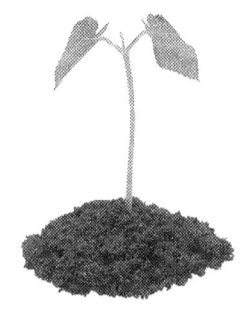

Part I
What Really Happened?

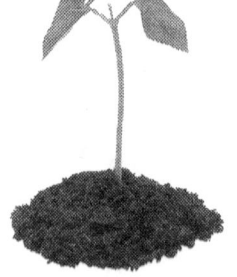

1
A Rare Disease Hits

What a piece of work is a man! How noble in reason! How infinite in faculties! In form and moving, how express and admirable!
—William Shakespeare; *Hamlet*

June 28 was a day my family will never forget. On a Sunday morning about a month earlier, my wife Sylvia and I were playing golf at Priddis Greens Golf and Country Club. The course was about fourteen years old and a future site of one of the year's top LPGA tournaments. It was wonderfully situated in the pristine country at the foothills of the Rocky Mountains just fifteen minutes by car from the western city limits of Calgary. We had been members since its first full season and had become accustomed to walking eighteen holes of the somewhat mountainous course at least twice a week in the golfing season. On this occasion, as was usual for a Sunday morning, our friends Bill and Reta finished out the foursome. We enjoyed working hard to improve our respective games and had a lot of fun doing it. As we made our way up the fairway on the eighteenth hole, Sylvia and I broke the news of our upcoming trip to Europe. We would not be able to golf for the next three weeks, but we gladly accepted Bill's offer to book us a time for the weekend following our return.

We finished the game, compared scores, traded excuses, changed into street shoes, and made our way to the car. Reta later recalled that as we walked across the parking lot, she experienced a cold feeling and had the rather ominous thought: *We will not be seeing them again.*

A First Step

I recall having had a 'chesty' cough. There were several nasty infections circulating around the office, including infectious viral pneumonia, signs of which, it was rumoured, did not show up on x-rays. Just to be safe, I decided to pay my family doctor a visit. I mentioned our upcoming trip to Europe. After a thorough going over, the doctor told me there was no indication of pneumonia. "Go and enjoy your holidays," he said. "The sun and warmth are probably just what you need." Much relieved, I made my way home and assured Sylvia that we could go on our trip as planned.

The date for departure arrived, and our daughter Ruth volunteered to drive us to the airport. It was during the drive that I realised I was not feeling well. The last thing I wanted was to be sick while away from home. We were walking over the pedestrian bridge leading to the terminal when I mentioned to Sylvia that perhaps we should think of postponing the trip. As soon as I had uttered the word 'postpone' and saw the reaction it created, I felt I was being rather selfish and wished I had bitten my tongue. One of the reasons for visiting England was to see Sylvia's brother Colin, who was terminally ill with cancer. *The doctor said the trip would do me good*, I told myself, *so no second thoughts. Let's just go. A decent holiday is what I need.*

Sylvia's other brother Jeff and his wife Sheila met us at Manchester Airport and, from that time on, totally spoiled us. For the next few days we were wined, dined, and generously accommodated. I excused my feeling off-colour, telling myself it was just jet lag. As soon as we were able, we arranged a visit with Colin and his wife Edith. They were more than happy to see us. In spite of his condition, Colin proved to be an excellent host, even to bringing out the cream cakes, which he remembered had been one of Sylvia's favourite treats as a child.

A day or two later, Jeff, Sheila, Sylvia and I joined up with Sylvia's sister Kath and her husband Jim. We visited the Liverpool Docks. The area we toured, which was close to the world-famous Liver Building, housed just about everything that made this port city famous, from models of Cunard Line ships, including the Titanic, to Beatles memorabilia. As we walked by the water's edge, there was a steady westerly wind. It was cool-sixteen or seventeen degrees Centigrade

— but in spite of wearing a thick woollen sweater and a golf jacket over my t-shirt, I couldn't get warm.

The next day, our hosts arranged a pub lunch, this time at the invitation of their son Ian and his wife Anne, who later invited us to their home. Still unnaturally cold, when we went out to their garden, I recall trying to find a spot in the sun. John brought out his soccer ball, and we kicked it around. I think I must have been England's star goalkeeper, at least in his sister Emma's opinion, if not in John's.

Another surprise awaited us. For our last evening, our hosts had arranged for the whole family to have a wonderful meal at a local country club, where we were able to create an enjoyable evening for Colin, who was understandably on everyone's mind.

The next day, we sadly took our leave of him, bade the rest of the family farewell, and made our way to Nottingham, where we visited cousin Janet and her husband, Bryan. There again, the welcome mat was out for us. We got to spend some time with Janet's sons Gary and Stuart, their friends Caroline and Mandy (wedding bells were to come later!), cousin Hilary, and her daughter Sally. The next day, after taking lots of photographs and enjoying a wonderful send-off lunch, Sylvia and I drove to Heathrow Airport to return our rental car. We soon ran into driving rain; but as we neared our destination, the clouds rolled back and the sun thankfully reappeared. I had forgotten how much rain could fall in England and was glad I would not have to unpack the car in a downfall.

After returning the car, we took a taxi to an old hotel on the outskirts of London and proceeded to try to get warm. Even though it was June, the rooms were damp and chilly. Later that evening, in view of my still not feeling one hundred per cent, Sylvia and I discussed the possibility of cutting our holiday short. As things stood, we would fly to Majorca, Spain, the following day. We talked it through and again decided to continue on, thinking that I would benefit from the warmer climate.

In the main, it was probably the right decision. We enjoyed temperatures in the upper twenties most of the time. I felt better in the warmth, but was running low on cough medicine, which had a particular ingredient that I would have to try to track down in the local pharmacies.

One morning we took a ferry to Port de Pollenca. Sylvia took advantage of a seat, and I took up a standing position at the bow to get a good view. It must have been close to thirty degrees Centigrade, but as the ferry left the dock and headed into the wind, I felt cold. It was an especially weird feeling, since I knew it was a hot day; but my body was not reacting as it should, and I had to withdraw to the cabin.

When we docked in Port de Pollenca, like most tourists, we headed for the shopping area hoping that, along with souvenirs, we could find a pharmacy where I could get my medication. There was, of course, the problem of a language barrier. Translating the ingredients of a medicine was not easy. In spite of our efforts, we had no luck-at least as far as the medication was concerned. Not so for souvenirs, however. Merchants at the port must have been pleased to see us coming.

Altogether, it was an enjoyable day. Sylvia loved the sea and the boating experience. She would have liked to take more trips on the ocean, but did not pursue the subject out of concern for the unusual feelings I was experiencing.

We spent the next few days on the beach relaxing in the sun. On our last day in the Cap de Formentor area, we packed our belongings and ordered a taxi to Palma de Mallorca, where we had planned an overnight stopover. The scenery was breathtaking! From the switchback, we had a wonderful view of the ocean. Upon leaving the coast, we settled back to enjoy the picturesque countryside with its quaint towns and villages.

When we reached our hotel in Palma, we settled in and ordered supper from room service. I was still not feeling right, though I could not put my finger on the problem and imagined it had to have something to do with my chest infection and the lack of medication, which by this time I'd been without for a few days. I was pleased we were finally on our way home, where I would be able to get a check up.

I did not need much persuading to make it an early night. Our Iberia flight to Barcelona was due to leave at 7:20 AM, and we had to be at the airport two hours before flight time.

··· *A Rare Disease Hits* ···

The wake-up call seemed to come almost as soon as I had gone to sleep. I was less then thrilled to catch a five AM taxi. The day stretched endlessly before me. With plane changes in Barcelona and a four-and-a-half hour layover at Heathrow, it would be twenty hours or so before we got home. I was greatly relieved to finally be taking off for Calgary. I had felt pretty well on the Spanish leg of the journey, but without my medication, I was coughing a lot.

I managed to catch some sleep on the plane and vividly recall the warmth of the fine summer afternoon that greeted Sylvia and I upon our textbook landing at Calgary International Airport. The next day, I went into the office, but by lunchtime jet lag was getting the better of me, so I decided to go home and take it a little easy, engaging in more restful pastimes, such as weeding the garden and cutting the lawn. The next two days were uneventful, and I was busy doing all the things one must do to catch up after returning from a holiday trip. I also paid a visit to my family doctor, who sent me for an x-ray, which later would prove to be clear.

The following morning-our first Sunday back home-dawned bright and clear and full of promise. We had planned to play golf, but it wasn't to be. I got out of bed to visit the washroom, took two steps, and collapsed. My legs simply gave way underneath me. I tried to get up, but was unable to do so until Sylvia, with superhuman strength, got me back on the bed. What had happened? I didn't know. *Was it a stroke*, I wondered? *No it couldn't be, could it? Surely it must be the flu; but then legs don't give way in cases of the flu.*

Sylvia's first reaction was to call for an ambulance. *Wait a minute*, I thought. *Surely there must be a simple explanation for what is happening to me.* I wanted to talk about it before making a big deal out of things, but the realization that this was something serious was slowly sinking in. Reluctantly, I agreed that she should make the call and settled back to wait for the paramedics.

Sylvia however had quite a different recollection. As she remembered it, not only was that day not sunny, it was, in fact, raining so hard that it was obvious the golf foursome arranged with our friends would be cancelled. We are all golf fanatics, but there are limits! Sylvia recalls allowing me to sleep in until early afternoon-in itself unusual. She then gave me brunch in bed and left me to rest a little longer. She was watering plants in an adjacent room when she heard a loud crash and rushed in to find me on the floor. Although I was amazed that she was able to get me back in bed, she later exclaimed that I appeared to be as light as a feather. It was as though she had somehow been able to draw on unknown reserves.

When I gave her a hard time about calling for an ambulance, she argued with me and then decided to call our eldest daughter Ruth, who came straight away, summed up the situation for herself, and took control from a very scared and distracted Sylvia.

Sylvia later related how shocked she was that this could happen to me. She obviously knew how fit I was, how I had always taken care of myself and been very fastidious in relation to health, exercising regularly and walking, even on the coldest days of winter.

Very soon the paramedics arrived and loaded me into the ambulance for the trip to Rockyview Hospital's emergency department. I remember the view through the rear window. It was a beautiful day, and I couldn't help feeling that nothing serious could be wrong. This thinking was encouraged when one of the paramedics commented that it did not appear to be a stroke, as both left and right sides were affected equally. A minute or two later, however, my heart fell. My reflexes, normally so strong they'd almost kick the doctor off his chair, were showing absolutely no response. "Looks like a neurological problem," said one paramedic. Sylvia later admitted wondering where we would go from here.

A young doctor examined me and told Sylvia he thought I had Guillain-Barré Syndrome (pronounced; ghee-yan/bah-ray). I vaguely remember his examination, but not his diagnosis. He suggested an immediate transfer to the Foothills Hospital, since they had a specialist who was familiar with GBS, as Guillain-Barré Syndrome is sometimes called.

An hour or so after we got to the Foothills, my diagnosis of generic GBS was confirmed. Further exclusionary testing was needed, though, to rule out additional rare things.

By this time, our daughters Ruth, Kim, and Sally had joined Sylvia. They were all struggling with the reality of my being diagnosed with something that was both rare and severe. To say they were shocked and frightened at my condition would be an understatement. It was such a blessing for Sylvia to have the family around for support. She had been so focused on my condition, it wasn't until we'd been in the Foothills Hospital for four hours that she looked down at her feet and noticed she was still wearing slippers.

Ruth was feeling alone too, as her husband Mark, who would have been very supportive, was overseas. She kept reassuring my wife that I would be all right. "This is Dad, so strong and able."

At this time I still had little understanding of just how serious my condition was. I never thought for one moment I would not be home again within a few days or a week at the very worst. I later learned that the news of my illness had really shaken my work associates and friends. I can hear most reactions now: "Guillain-Barré Syndrome, what's that?" When I first heard the diagnosis, I did not even know how to pronounce the name, never mind spell it.

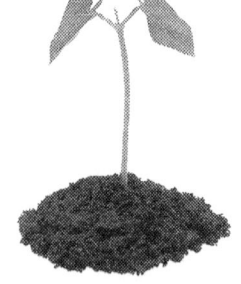

2
What Is This Disorder?

The historical background of this syndrome is interesting, and has a place here.

The disorder commonly called Guillain-Barré (ghee-yan/bah-ray) syndrome is a rare illness that affects the peripheral nerves of the body. Its main feature is weakness, and even paralysis, often accompanied by abnormal sensations. The syndrome occurs sporadically. It can't be predicted, and can occur at any age and in either sex. It can vary greatly in severity from the mildest case that may not even be brought to a doctor's attention, to a devastating illness with almost complete paralysis that brings a patient close to death. Because it is so rare, most of the public has never heard of the illness, or if they have, know little about it. Yet, for those affected, the illness can be severely disabling.[1]

The term syndrome, rather than disease, is used to describe the illness observed by Guillain and others. This term reflects the recognition of the illness by the collection of symptoms (what the patient tells the physician about changes in his body) and signs (what the doctor observes upon examining the patient) that typify the disorder.[2]

In 1859, a French physician, Jean B. O. Landry, described in detail a disorder of the nerves that paralyzed the legs, arms, neck and breathing muscles of the chest. Several reports of a similar disorder followed from other countries. The demonstration by Quinke in 1891, of spinal fluid removal by passing a needle into the low back, paved the way for three Parisian physicians, Georges Guillain, Jean Alexander Barré and Andre Strohl to show, in 1916, the characteristic abnormality of increased fluid protein with normal cell count.[3]

These three French doctors were working at the time

...in the Sixth Army Hospital Unit when two serving soldiers were admitted just after the Battle of the Somme with paralysis. One of these patients was an infantryman who on attempting to put on his backpack fell backwards with its weight and was unable to rise again. Their examination of this soldier included a graphical record of his knee reflexes which showed that muscle reflex movements were considerably delayed.[4]

Guillain and his co-workers correctly deduced that the primary problem lay within the peripheral nerves and not as Landry had assumed within the central nervous system. They also drew attention to the cerebrospinal fluid findings which have ever since been used to help confirm the diagnosis of GBS. The CSF contained a raised level of protein with out any evidence of extra white cells usually found in inflammatory conditions common at that time such as syphilis or tuberculosis. Guillain, Barré and Strohl's report left the question of the cause of the disease open assuming that it must be an intoxification or an infection.[5]

Treatment in those days was much more interesting than it is today. While Landry treated his patient with injections of strychnine (unsuccessfully as it turned out), Guillain and colleagues used chops and Bordeaux wine which were extremely efficacious since (their two) patients recovered quickly. Indeed Guillain maintained all his life that GBS was a mild illness and that fatal cases like that of Landry must really be a different disease.[6]

Since then, several investigators have collected additional information about this disorder. It can affect nerves not only to the limbs and breathing muscles, but also those to the throat, heart, urinary bladder and eyes. Doctors have several names for the syndrome, including acute [rapid onset of] inflammatory [irritated], polyneuropathy [disease of many nerves], acute idiopathic [of unknown cause], polyneuritis [irritation or inflammation of many nerves], acute idiopathic polyradiculoneuritis, Landry's ascending paralysis, acute dysimmune [to reflect the probably abnormal immune or protective response by the body against its own nerves that Guillain-Barré syndrome represents] polyneuropathy [disease of many nerves], etc. If full credit were to be given to those physicians who first recognized and described the paralyzing disorder that we now commonly call Guillain-Barré Syndrome, or GBS, then its name might properly be Landry-Guillain-Barré-Strohl Syndrome. But, alas, Drs. Landry and Strohl are usually forgotten.[7]

What is Guillain-Barré Syndrome?[8]

When we decide to perform some activity, such as walking, the brain sends an electric signal down a nerve path in the spinal cord [in the back], and this signal, in turn, is conducted out of the spinal cord by nerves that go to our muscles [an example is the sciatic nerve to the legs]. The latter nerves, those that extend from the spinal cord outwards, are called peripheral nerves. These are the nerves that are damaged in GBS. They extend outwards from the spinal cord to the limbs, chest muscles of respiration, internal organs [heart, etc.] and so forth. Some of those nerves are covered, much as are electric wires in our home, by insulation. The insulation covering of nerves is called myelin [my-eh-lin]. In GBS, the myelin or insulation is damaged. This damage seems to slow down or short circuit the ability of the nerve to conduct a signal normally. With the slowed signal conduction, patients experience weakness. If conduction is too slow, or even blocked, the patient may become paralyzed. The nerve insulation surrounds a central conducting core or wire, called the axon [axé-ahn]. The development of long-term paralysis in some GBS patients may reflect permanent damage of not only the nerve's myelin insulation but also its central conducting core or axon.

The peripheral nerves affected in GBS include, not only the motor nerves that extend from the spinal cord to muscles, but also the sensory nerves that extend from the skin, muscles, and joints to the cord, and send signals about our surroundings to the cord and then brain. These sensory nerves allow us to feel temperature, limb position, coarse and smooth fabric surfaces, etc. When they are damaged in GBS, the patient experiences decreased or even abnormal sensations.

In GBS, not only the nerves to and from the limbs are affected. Nerves from the spinal cord to the chest muscles used for respiration are also affected. In addition, the nerves to and from the internal organs, heart, bowel, etc., can be involved. These are the nerves of the automatic [or, in medical language, the autonomic] nervous system.

As described above, in GBS, the myelin covering of nerves is damaged, and, in severe cases, even the enclosed nerve axon can be damaged. Another variant of GBS, more common in China, has also been described in which the nerve core or axon is damaged, but with myelin coating remaining intact, so-called axonal GBS. These patients often do poorly.

In GBS, the brain and spinal cord do not appear to be affected. Thus, functions of the brain and some of the short nerves coming out of it, for example, to the ears and nose, are preserved. Patients can usually think, hear and smell normally.[9]

* * *

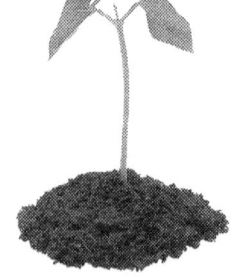

3
What Causes Guillain-Barré Syndrome?

One of the most frequently asked questions on the subject of Guillain-Barré Syndrome, once the disorder is described and understood, is about the cause. That is discussed here.

What Causes Guillain-Barré Syndrome?[10]
　　The cause of Guillain-Barré syndrome is not known. A variety of events seem to trigger the illness. Many cases occur a few days to a few weeks after a viral infection. These infections include the common cold, sore throat, and stomach and intestinal illnesses with diarrhea. Some cases have been associated with specific infectious agents. [These include cytomegalovirus, Epstein-Barr virus (that causes infectious mononucleosis), Mycoplasma pneumoniae, and the gram negative bacterium found in the bowel, Campylobacter jejuni/coli.] However, the mechanism(s) by which these microorganisms may lead to GBS has not yet been determined. Some cases have occurred with a rare disease of red blood cells, porphyria. Some GBS-like cases have occurred after such seemingly unrelated events as surgery, insect stings and various injections. Many cases occurred in the Winter of 1976–77 in persons who received the swine flu vaccine.

A few outbreaks or clusters of GBS or GBS-like disorders have been reported, including summer epidemics in rural northern Chinese children, a Jordanian outbreak in 1978 upon exposure to polluted water, and an outbreak in Finland after a nationwide oral poliovirus vaccination campaign. The stomach bacterium, Campylobacter jejeuni, has been implicated as a triggering factor in the Chinese paralytic syndrome; in other clusters the cause has not become evident.

It is of interest that literally millions of people have been exposed to events, such as infections, surgery, and vaccines that have been identified as triggering agents for GBS. Yet only a very small number of people exposed to these events develop GBS. Why only certain people develop GBS is unclear. Might they have some unique genetic predisposition? Since it is rare for more than one member of a family to develop GBS, it seems unlikely that a genetic factor plays a significant role. Hopefully further research will improve our understanding of how and why GBS occurs.

Research to date indicates that, regardless of the triggering event, the nerves of the Guillain-Barré patient are attacked by the body's own defense system against disease-antibodies and white blood cells. As a result of this autoimmune attack, the nerve insulation (myelin) and sometimes even the covered conducting part of the nerve (axon) is damaged and signals are delayed or otherwise changed. Abnormal sensations and weakness follow.

One currently proposed mechanism to explain how GBS develops in some patients involves the concept of molecules that look alike or mimic each other (molecular mimicry), with the nerve becoming damaged as an innocent bystander. According to this explanation, some of the molecules in an infecting bug or other substance, e.g., bacteria, virus, immunization, etc., are quite similar to some of the molecules in myelin or other parts of the nerve. When such foreign material enters the body, as with an infection, it triggers the patient's immune defense system to mount an attack against that invader. If some of the infecting bug's molecules look like or mimic myelin or other nerve molecules, the patient's immune system recognizes not only the invading bug as foreign, but also mistakenly recognizes the nerve as foreign, and attacks both. Thus, because some of the nerve molecules look like or mimic those of the invader, the nerve is incorrectly identified by the patient's immune system as foreign, and becomes an innocent bystander that is inadvertently or accidentally attacked and injured. In other words, to the patient's immune defence system, both the invading bug (e.g., infecting bacteria, etc.) and part of the patient's own nerves look alike, so both are attacked. Mounting evidence supports this mechanism to explain why some people who are exposed to the stomach bacterium, Campylobacter jejuni, develop GBS or a similar disorder. Ongoing research may help to decipher in what cases of GBS this mechanism occurs, so that perhaps treatments can be developed to reduce or prevent the accidental nerve damage.

Because Guillain-Barré syndrome often follows a viral illness, it is sometimes mistakenly thought to be contagious. However, there is no evidence that it can be caught, even if a person had contact with the patient during the preceding viral infection. In fact, often the virus is no longer in the patient when the syndrome is developing.[11]

In my case, the cause was never established. I have heard it claimed that, in addition to causes already mentioned, flu vaccinations other than that for the swine flu and even tick bites could be responsible. I believe it has to be recognized, though, that the risk of contracting GBS through an influenza vaccination is extremely remote. The flu shot has to be seen as a lifesaver-and just for the record, I had suffered the indignity of a tick bite five years prior. I recall finding the tick and, following timeworn advice, tried unsuccessfully to burn it out. I ended up at the Emergency Room of our local hospital, where it was safely removed. I asked the doctor if there were any warning signs that I should be aware of. I had Lyme disease or Rocky Mountain spotted fever in mind. His reply surprised me. He said that if I experienced any paralysis in my lower extremities, I should get to the ER quickly. I now believe he was describing the onset of Guillain-Barré Syndrome.

One thing that intrigues me is that a number of other patients with whom I have spoken had been traveling overseas or had recently returned when GBS struck. This raised the question of a possible "travel connection". I am not convinced there isn't one, although I can't speculate on whether the virus responsible for my infection was picked up overseas or if, perhaps, it was triggered at a time when my immune system was compromised by jet lag.

Having learned the part that the immune system plays in the devastating onset of this disease, and knowing how fit and healthy I was at the time of its onset, I am convinced that the stronger a person's immune system, the more severe the case. This theory- although not one most medical professionals like to admit-would provide a reason for my developing the 'severe acute chronic axonal' variant of Guillain-Barré Syndrome.

Even if true, however, I would never discourage anyone from aiming for anything short of total fitness. If you were unfortunate enough to be one of the few afflicted by Guillain-Barré Syndrome, being otherwise fit would enable you to better fight the actual infection and all the subsequent infections you might encounter. I am sure my fitness helped me to win the battle against it. Without my high level of fitness, this story might have had a different ending.

...

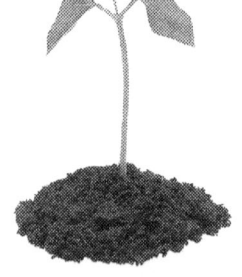

4
Destination: Intensive Care

I was not aware of being transferred from the ER to Intensive Care at the Foothills Hospital in Calgary. What little memory I have of this period is spotty. Fortunately, my wife had the foresight, and perhaps also the need, to put her thoughts on paper. She had been devastated, not only by my diagnosis, but by the speed of the syndrome's progress. I went from being a normal, healthy person, albeit with a respiratory infection in common with other associates at that time, to a helpless, totally paralysed individual with a dismal prognosis.

The onset of my paralysis was fairly sudden. I was not aware of its specific progress, but knew I could not stand up. I believe from all accounts that the paralysis began in my feet and legs and traveled up my body, eventually reaching my chest and lungs, then moved into my shoulders, arms, neck, and face, finally halting just above my eyebrows. This all happened within the space of forty-eight hours.

Sylvia's initial notes, which were undated, but I believe relate to June 30, two days after admission, indicated I was already on a ventilator. I had lost the ability to speak, and communicated by raising or lowering my forehead. A straight face indicated 'no'; a raised forehead meant 'yes.' She noted I had kept my sense of humour. One of my first requests was to ask if someone could rub my feet.

Later in the day, I must have regained the use of my eyebrows, as the signalling code was changed to one blink for a 'no' and two for a 'yes'. Invariably either the nurses or I would get the code

··· *A First Step* ···

mixed up, and that led to confusion and frustration, particularly if I tried to make a joke. Panic could ensue.

I should have known better. In my condition, how could I expect the nursing staff to believe I was joking or making light of something? Yet when an opportunity presented itself, I could not resist.

On that same day, Sylvia noted that morphine had been administered, in addition to a two-hour treatment of immuno-gamma globulin. Overnight, my white blood count rose. July 1 dawned, and I had one of many x-rays. I was given insulin to keep my blood sugar down, and I was moved to a private room. Four days after admission, a single line entry in her journal included that much-dreaded word 'pneumonia'. Bacterial pneumonia set in on July 2. My left lung was badly infected, and a battle for survival appears to have ensued. A diagnostic technique known as *bronchoalveolar lavage* was utilized to identify which bugs I had. Thankfully, although it was bad enough, staphylococcus aureus was not one of the really bad drug-resistant strains. It was, therefore, possible to follow with a course of antibiotics. As was to be expected, my blood pressure was up and down. I managed to move my chin, or was it imagined? I did have movement in my eyebrows. That fit the pattern. I later learned that the last muscles to go down in GBS are usually the first to come back.

During this time, my immediate family was exhausted from the long hours spent with me in Intensive Care and from the stress of worry. The support they received from friends, my business colleagues, other family members, and the nursing staff will long be remembered.

The day of the world famous Calgary Stampede Parade came and went. Sylvia recorded it in the journal as being a wet day, which was most unusual, since it never rains on the parade, or so legend has it. She and our daughter Ruth spent most of the day watching over me. I had experienced a reasonable night and, after being suctioned three times, appeared more comfortable and alert. I was again able to show off movement in my eyebrows and chin. My hands and feet were now in braces to keep them straight and to avoid drooping. The family was encouraged to gently exercise both areas.

The doctor, pleased to see me feeling a little better, decided to sit me in a wheelchair for half an hour. In her journal, Sylvia wrote, *This was awful to see; he was so helpless- no control at all, but once they padded him up, he looked comfy.* Other signs-heart and blood pressure-were good. The antibiotics seemed to be doing their job. Late in the day when my daughter Sally came to visit, she was able to lip-read my enquiry as to how she and her family were. That I could move my lips had everyone pretty excited.

I believe I owe a special thanks to Vi and all the other nurses in Intensive Care at the Foothills Hospital and at Rockyview Hospital, where my stay was much longer. Although I can't remember it, I'm told that on the fourth of July they gave me a shave, complete with aftershave lotion. Vi, especially, was a pillar of strength and provided wonderful support to the family. Later that morning I had my tracheotomy done, and was seen moving my chin again. More fluid was taken from my lungs.

After a reasonable night, I spent a short time in the wheelchair and asked for a drink of water. My request was, of course, denied. I could not swallow anything and was being fed intravenously. More than four months would pass before I would be able to savour a clear, cool glass of water. The immediate problem was partially solved, however, by the duty nurse, who used mouthwash sponges to moisten and refresh my mouth.

I had short sessions of physiotherapy (PT) and occupational therapy (OT); and, the doctor seemed reasonably satisfied with my progress. Later though, the nurse became concerned about my heart rate, which appeared to be getting uneven. After another suction, however, the rate steadied and things settled down.

Since there were only two small windows in the intensive care unit, the lights were on all day. I had no regular meal times because of the intravenous feeding, so there was concern that I would become disoriented. It was now July 7, and the pneumonia was still being cleared. It was very warm and I was taken outside in a wheelchair for a five-minute walk, all padded up so as not to fall over. Not surprisingly, I found the sun very bright and needed sunglasses.

I guess it was hard for anyone witnessing my transfer from bed to chair and back. My head was very unstable. In fact, I had no control. Sylvia thought she recognized some new facial movement, though.

A family conference was called for the next day, at which time one of the doctors explained about how Guillain-Barré Syndrome was affecting me and the treatment, including receiving gamma globulin over the course of five days, to be repeated if needed.

Apparently, I did not sleep well and was convinced that Foothills had lost me overnight. "How did you find me?" was my question to Sylvia, Ruth, and Mark when they came visiting that morning. It was the first of many dreams I was to experience in which it was difficult, if not impossible, to distinguish the dream world from reality. In subsequent dreams and hallucinations, I had almost total recall down to the smallest detail.

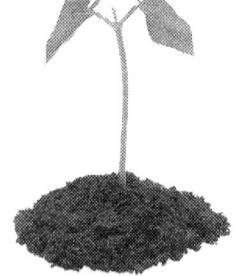

5
New Quarters
...

The morning of July 10 saw me stable enough to be transferred to Rockyview General Hospital in Calgary. The reason, as I later learned, was that although the Foothills Medical Centre was the regional centre for trauma, neurosurgery, and cardiovascular surgery, resources were scarce. They had run out of ICU beds and had to transfer someone to the Peter Lougheed Centre or Rockyview, the other two facilities in the city. Luckily, Rockyview was convenient for my family. The environment there was completely different. Although I was still in the ICU, I had a very pleasant view of the woodland bordering the Glenmore Reservoir. Under other circumstances, one might well have imagined being in a resort hotel. Later that morning, early visitors found me in good shape and sleeping normally. My blood sugar was up a little, and Sylvia was happy to see me grimace and really move my chin in response to one of her comments.

Here is what Sylvia wrote in her diary regarding my progress subsequent to my transfer to Rockyview:

> **July 11**
> *S. Diary* Brian's second day at Rockyview. He's feeling more comfortable and has pictures from home around him. I was with him most of the day and was able to take him for a short walk outside in a wheelchair. Getting him into the chair was no mean feat, and it took six or seven nurses to transfer him from the bed.

... A First Step ...

Brian is not comfortable in the chair. He needs a tabletop for his arms and more support for his head. He also complains of discomfort in his feet. Morphine helps.

July 12
S. Diary Brian had a reasonably comfortable night. Son-in-law Dwayne fixed up a TV and VCR. The doctor reduced the ventilator from twelve breaths a minute to nine. Brian moved his face more, had good colour, and not quite so much suction was needed.

July 13
S. Diary Things were a little uneasy today. There was some discomfort from the tracheotomy.

July 15
S. Diary The ventilator is now down to eight breaths a minute, and Brian takes four breaths a minute on his own. This tires him out and is probably what makes it hard to get any answers from him.

July 16
S. Diary Brian was in his wheelchair for an hour and a half, but this time with a neck brace. He was not very cheerful and seemed even to be sad. Sally talked to the neuro specialist, who wanted him back on immuno gamma globulin to help boost his immune system.

July 17
S. Diary Things are looking much better. The neck brace has created some discomfort and is going to be altered or, if necessary, remade. For now, Brian is free of any distress, and I left him comfortable and watching the British Open.

July 19

S. Diary Brian should have had EMG tests today, but they were put off until Wednesday. He is communicating much more with his eyebrows and is trying to smile.

July 20

S. Diary Daughter Kim visited this evening.

July 21

S. Diary The results of Brian's tests came in today. They are bad. In a nutshell, he has a severe case of GBS The family is in shock. The prognosis is worse than anyone expected. I never dreamt it would be so awful. Now I am scared. A meeting has been arranged for Friday to answer the family's questions. Let's hope we get answers that will enable us to tell Brian he has reason to hope.

July 23

S. Diary Pam Barnie was Brian's nurse today. I gave his arms a massage, trying to give him strength. In spite of everything, he is in fairly good spirits.

July 24

S. Diary We had the family meeting this afternoon. The doctor did not dwell on the results disclosed on Wednesday. Instead, he promised Brian would be re-tested in a few weeks. Right now, he insists we must keep ourselves very fit and involve Brian with the household bills, local and world news, sports news, and the stock market to keep his mind alert. We adopted a visiting plan whereby Ruth, Kim, Sally, Brian's brother Roger and his wife Stella, and I would take turns, allowing for all of us to have some time off.

July 25

S. Diary Very hot today-28 degrees Centigrade. Brian seemed to be very comfortable. The eyebrow movement was there, and the nurse, Loverna, had him up in the wheelchair for a while, complete with a modified neck brace. The new brace didn't appear to be causing him any discomfort. There was no contact with the doctors, but I could not help feeling easier in the knowledge he has a second chance. Hopefully, in the next four to six weeks there will be some improvement.

July 26

S. Diary After experiencing a restless night, Brian was very comfortable and relaxed this afternoon. I thought his tongue looked more natural and hope it wasn't just my imagination.

July 27

S. Diary Today was Brian's birthday. The family did a great job decorating his room. It looked pretty all decked out with cards and balloons. Sally brought in a cake, and except for Brian, we all-including staff-enjoyed it. Everyone joined in to sing 'Happy Birthday'. It was a tough day for Brian. His heart rate was a little uneven and, by the time we left him, he was very tired and had just fallen asleep.

July 28

S. Diary This was my day off. I played golf at Priddis Greens with our friends Bill and Reta. Had a good day, played a good game, and felt really refreshed. The golf pro, Tim, asked to be remembered to Brian. Everyone there misses him and wishes him well.

July 29

S. Diary Had a call from the Rockyview. The doctor wanted to see me at 11:00 AM I arrived to be told that, after testing for blood in the urine, Brian has a cancerous tumour and they have decided to operate in two days. My poor husband! How much more can he take? He must be so worried, and he can't even talk to us about it.

July 30

S. Diary They gave Brian two pints of blood in preparation for tomorrow's operation. He seemed to be having a good day. The nurses thought he looked great. The ventilator setting was 6 breaths per minute, or BPM, and Brian was breathing himself at the rate of 11 BPM Thank goodness we don't have to wait until next week for the results of his surgery.

July 31

S. Diary Brian was operated on at the Rockyview General Hospital. All went well. Thank goodness, they were mistaken about the cancer. The culprits were bladder stones, which they removed. I was just so relieved to be given that news and immediately phoned the family. What a great result!

Aug 1

S. Diary After the operation, Brian had a reasonable night. His heart rate was up a little-a sign of pain-but otherwise he rested okay. Kim and Buck came by. Brian was a little distressed, but I think that was his reaction to yesterday's operation when the possibility of cancer existed. Later in the day, his heart rate fell, but it came back on its own. The doctor thought he did well today, but I thought he seemed tired.

Aug 2
S. Diary A good day. Brian was really using his chin, trying hard to say 'yes'. Sally and I were with him for nearly three hours.

Aug 3
S. Diary Sally and I visited during the morning for a change. We decided afternoons were far better. Brian was much the same.

Aug 4
S. Diary A much better day. Brian's ventilator was set at 6 BPM His nurse did not appear too impressed, but we were.

Aug 5
S. Diary I had a day off and played golf; then paid some bills, which I find very stressful. Brian used to take care of this. I keep wondering how things will end.

Aug 6
S. Diary Brian was up for about twenty minutes with the neck brace on. He didn't look too comfortable, but it is better for him. Good colour again, and he tried to smile. Not much change in the overall picture, though. There is still a very long way to go.

Aug 7
S. Diary They are trying something new to help Brian get his voice back. The doctor thought he noticed stronger neck movement.

Aug 8
S. Diary Telephone call from the hospital-the Doctor wanted to change the position of Brian's feeding tube from his nose to his stomach. I gave the necessary

consent. It would make Brian more comfortable. He sat up in the wheelchair for forty-five minutes, and they plan to increase the time each day.

Aug 9

S. Diary Brian seemed much brighter and was glad to see us. He was much more comfortable in bed. Later, due to the staff being busy with an emergency elsewhere in the hospital, he had to stay in his chair nearly two-and-a- quarter hours. By the end of that, he looked stressed.

Aug 10

S. Diary Kim, Roger, and I visited. A chest x-ray was done. Peggy, his nurse for the day, seemed quite happy with his progress.

Aug 11

S. Diary I saw Brian move his neck! What a great feeling. It is still early, we know, but it is wonderful to see his achievement.

Aug 12

S. Diary Another operation, this time to remove the feeding tube from his nose and replace it in his stomach. When Ruth and I were finally able to see him, he was very sleepy and, most of the time, didn't know us. We all, including the doctor, knew Brian was hurting. Eventually it was decided that he was hungry. He'd had no food since last night.

Aug 13

S. Diary Brian was up in his chair for about an hour. He still does not like the neck brace and seemed somewhat distressed about that and his tracheotomy site, which was leaking and had blood in it.

Aug 14

S. Diary I phoned the hospital at 9:30 this morning. Brian had been awake all night, and his tracheotomy site is still leaking. I am so sad for him. I can't imagine how he must feel. The family rallied around- Ruth and Mark dropped me off; then Kim and Buck took me home after supper. It has been a long day for all of us.

Aug 15

S. Diary Found Brian much more comfortable today. His colour was really good. The therapist did exercises while I was there, and I thought I noticed Brian move his left shoulder. I told his nurse. She was a little surprised, but the therapist agreed that he did move it once. He seems much more comfortable in his chair. For a change of scenery, he sat in the hallway for about an hour. The tracheotomy site has stopped leaking.

Aug 16

S. Diary Brian was hurting and Ruth and I had a hard time figuring out where. Called Pam in to help, and she discovered he was lying on his left ear and it was bent over. He could not move his head to help himself. Afterwards he was smiling at us quite a bit.

Aug 17

S. Diary The doctor told me not to get my hopes up too high regarding the new EMG test scheduled for the 19th. "The results may not be what we all want."

Aug 18

S. Diary Brian was up in his chair for an hour and twenty minutes, but he looked stressed at the end of it. Peggy is taking care of him today. He had good

··· New Quarters ···

head movement and was able to smile. I feel he is happy, and I'm going home to get some rest.

Aug 19

S. Diary   What an awful day! The EMG results were not good. They showed no nerve activity below the neck. Doctors now anticipate a recovery will take one to two years, and it is unlikely to be complete. Nerves grow about an inch a month, and it is anticipated they will take about a year to reach the diaphragm. They told me Brian would not be allowed to come home until he is able to breath on his own or with the aid of a ventilator if he can manage to adjust it himself. They are worried about possible complications-infection, pneumonia, bleeding ulcers, etc.

❊ ❊ ❊

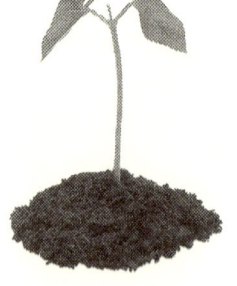

6
As Bad As It Gets

Almost two months after admission to the ER at the Foothills Hospital, the verdict was pronounced. It was not what anyone wanted to hear. Guillain-Barré Syndrome was confirmed, but in my case with the axonal degeneration variant. It could hardly be worse. This was not the garden variety of GBS

The news must have been much more devastating for Sylvia and the family than it was for me. At the time, I did not realize the full implications of the diagnosis, but merely sensed I had a fight on my hands. My vocabulary did not include the word 'defeat', and I just refused to believe I could not get my life back to normal, however long it might take. Certainly I could not talk, but as her diary indicated, Sylvia knew me well enough to recognize I was up to the challenge:

> **Aug 20**
> S. Diary   Brian is concerned about the possibility of being sent home with a respirator and wondering how it would be arranged. Mark was able to make him understand that it would be taken care of. The doctor was good with us. He seemed to understand how we felt, as did Peggy, the nurse. She was very sympathetic. Through much of what went on, Brian was smiling, seemingly trying to tell us he knows that he has a long struggle to face and he is up to it.

Aug 21

S. Diary   We are trying out a new wheelchair. It is very light and easy to move. Brian looked all right in it, but needs the headrest adjusted and more space for his legs. He went outside for fifteen minutes, but was very tired afterwards. Seven nurses were needed to put him back to bed-three positioned themselves on the bed, one held his head to keep it stable, and three lifted him from the chair. It looked so straightforward, but what if we hurt him again?

Aug 22

S. Diary   A depressing day. Our patient was very uncomfortable. The nurse, Flo, did what she could to help. Brian had some trouble breathing, but he appears to be trying to swallow, which is a positive thing. He has not been sleeping well. Last night it was 4 AM before he fell asleep, and then it was only for two hours. Flo bathed him and manicured his hands and feet. Sally and I stayed about two hours and left feeling quite guilty. Apparently, the heart rate and blood pressure reading were good; otherwise they would be concerned.

Aug 23

S. Diary   Sally, Dwayne, and I went in again to find Brian in his chair. This was a much better day for him, and he had smiles for all of us. Mona was his nurse, and she was very sweet. She had shaved him and made him comfortable. At one point, I read the sports page to him and he fell asleep. Kim, Buck, and the boys drove me home after we had left the TV and VCR ready for the evening.

...

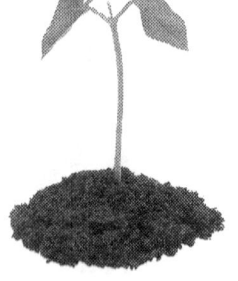

7
Patients and Their Televisions

I hoped all the good people who were concerned about me-nurses, family and friends-were not upset at my lack of interest in having a TV. I believe there were times when I must have appeared most ungrateful; but apart from news, sports, and our favourite, the PBS channel from Spokane, neither my wife nor I were addicts. To my surprise, even as I lay paralysed in a hospital bed, I was not particularly interested in television. It seemed a waste of time. Preferring my own memories and fantasy life, I spent hours recalling vacations, golf, and times spent with my family. I created a dream world of adventure and travel, and-of increasing importance as the months passed-I made plans. I mapped out a daily timetable for living once I was out of hospital, made mental lists of the people I wanted to see, and thought about the things I wanted to do.

At the time, communicating this information to others was far too complicated, so I just had to hope everyone understood that, in spite of my condition, I might well be the only patient in the hospital who did not need a TV for entertainment.

Perhaps a significant reason for this was I could not use my hands and could not, therefore, use the remote control. If, for example, someone were to leave me with a golf game on, the game would end and there I'd be stuck with a soap opera, in which I was not the least bit interested. I would have to suffer in silence until a nurse happened to drop in to turn the thing off.

Now back to Sylvia's description of my life on a ventilator:

Aug 24

S. Diary   Brian was in his chair when I arrived, but tired. Later I found the likely reason-his ventilator had been reduced to 4 BPM; so now he has to work his lung muscles harder than before. It will take a while for him to get used to it, but they are monitoring him closely.

Aug 25

S. Diary   The ventilator setting was back to 6 BPM Yesterday's setting of 4 BPM was too low, at least for the time being. He is looking good and communicating more clearly by nodding his head and raising his eyebrows. His chair now has a tray on the back to transport the respirator. He enjoyed an outside walk with me. I am getting better at lip-reading.

Aug 26

S. Diary   I took a break today. Sally visited Brian late in the day and noted his breathing aid was back down to 4 BPM

Aug 27

S. Diary   In his chair for an hour and a half, Brian looked much more like his usual self, although by the time they transferred him back to bed, he was quite tired. I hope this is a good sign. The ventilator is still set at 4 BPM, and he is doing 11 BPM on his own.

Aug 28

S. Diary   Today, the ventilator was set at a rate of only 1 BPM They are trying to wean him off it. I hope they are not rushing this just to get him in a medical ward. He appears to be worried about the ventilator setting, and I think he is upset at having to be in a chair; but if he wants to come home, he will have to do it. Never did we ever think this would be happening to us. A new doctor was on duty, and he reiterated that Brian's progress will be long and slow. Why do they keep telling us this? We know it, and being told over and over just increases our stress level.

Aug 29

S. Diary Today Brian was up in his chair for two hours, including a twenty-minute walk outside. His nurse Nancy Van Berkel was very good with him. He was pleased to see me, and we had a great visit. There was no reading on the ventilator screen for most of the time I was there. He was doing twelve BPM on his own. The nurse thought he was experiencing some shoulder pain, but we shall see. I am feeling pretty good today. I thank God for listening to my prayers. I think we have made a start in getting Brian back with us. He winked at me today with so much love in his eyes. Even his brother Roger, who was also visiting, said, "Look at that Sylvia."

Aug 31

S. Diary Mark leaves for China. Ruth will join him later for a holiday. The doctor said he saw some improvement and that he'd noticed Brian's shoulders beginning to move. Later Brian managed without a neck brace for half an hour, did neck exercises, and held his head up without support. He looked very happy at the achievement, and even his nurse was impressed.

We tried our best at lip-reading, but it creates so much stress that it's hard to leave him at the end of the day. In spite of that, I feel better about

... A First Step ...

Brian today. He kept giving us smiles as if to say, "Don't worry, I'm O.K."

Sept. 1

S. Diary Therapy has started. It seems electronic pulses are being used to stimulate Brian's shoulder and neck muscles. He is being kept up a little longer each day. He held up his head without a brace for a few minutes-looked unsteady, but seemed pleased with himself. Progress will be slow, but every step achieved is a plus. We know he is fighting.

Sept 2

S. Diary My day off. Sally visited Brian. It was a nice day, but there was definitely a fall feeling in the air.

Sept 3

S. Diary I feel like celebrating! Brian was really showing off his neck movements today. Everyone was impressed, including the nurses. There were a few moist eyes. Nurse Flo said she felt like crying. I know Ruth and I did.

Brian did not want us to touch his arms while he was exercising his neck, and when his therapist Margot Sondermann told him he had done great and should relax, he laughed his heart out. The room was full of people, all showing their support. The plan is to keep him up in the wheelchair for longer periods each day-three hours today.

Now that Brian can move his head, we are trying a new communication system. He has a cap with a pointer attached. Someone holds an alphabet board in front of him, and by moving his head he can spell out a message. So far it is working.

We still have a long way to go, but we have started.

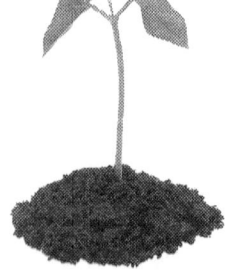

8
The Art & Importance of Communicating

...

By this time, everyone was becoming interested in my means of communication. Originally, I'd raise my eyebrows, once for a yes, twice for a no-or was it the other way around? Once I regained the ability to move my neck, it was possible to devise a system whereby I wore a baseball cap with a pointer affixed, and I would use my head to point to a word or letter on the word board.

Over time, our system expanded and whole sentences such as *I am uncomfortable*; *I am cold*; or *Can I have a suction?* were listed on the board. In his paper entitled *Communication and Altered Perceptions* published in New Jersey Medicine, Doctor Kopel Burk, who was himself a GBS patient, went one step further. He wrote:

> I began working with my daughter, Tina, on a better system: whole words and sentences on a single card. Our system was even more sophisticated, cards that were color-coded. Three sentences were on each card. Pink cards were for personal needs: *I'm in pain. I need the bed pan. Please move my arms or legs. Please wash my face.* Green cards were questions for the doctors: *How was my x-ray? How did the lab work come out?* Blue cards were general questions for my family: *Have you heard from Mark? How is Rachel? What's new in the world?*
>
> The top card in each of the color packs was iden-

tical: *Please show me the cards. I want to use the pink group, blue group, or green group.*

We added to the cards by using the alphabet board to identify new areas to cover. In about four days we had a whole communication system on color-coded cards.

In the same paper, Doctor Burk later describes his reaction to others with GBS two and a half years after his brush with the disease:

> Whenever I make rounds on the intensive care unit, I usually stop for a moment to watch the patients on respirators. Some of the patients are comatose. Others are awake, but seem confused and restless. An occasional patient, however, is alert and oriented.
>
> I look to see if there has been an attempt to make communication possible for this alert patient — the electronic board, the color-coded cards, or the Cooper-Rand speech device. If I find anything at all, it usually is a crudely drawn up alphabet chart. It is almost as if everyone is required to reinvent the wheel. When I ask about the use of the more sophisticated aids to help this patient communicate, I am told that the patient will be weaned from the respirator in a day or so. This answer suggests that in the priority list of acute medical care needs, communication is not at the top. For the short term ventilator patient, they might be correct. But anyone involved in the care of a long-term respirator patient or patients with a permanent speech defect should learn about the wide range of assistance in communication available in all hospitals.

Doctor Burk continued:

> Having been chairman of the Bioethics Commit-

tee of Overlook Hospital, I am committed to the concept that competent patients should be involved in making decisions regarding their medical care. Such a dialogue required input from physician and patient. When the patient is on a ventilator, that presents a challenge. Yet, I have been surprised to find that some patients on respirators are more successful at the art of communicating than are their physicians.[12]

Back to Sylvia's journal, and new worries:

Sept 4

S. Diary Had a meeting with the doctor and staff about Brian's condition. Progress is very slow, and he will be at Rockyview for months. He has three infections right now. It will be necessary to gown-up and wear gloves whenever entering his room. This applies to everyone-nurses, staff, and visitors alike. They are trying to set up regular groups of nurses so that everyone involved with him will know the objectives: time in chair, time outside, communicating with the aid of the baseball cap, and involvement in daily matters.

When I was asked how Brian must be feeling, I responded, "Scared and lonely; worried about being alone after we leave; fear of choking; worried about me; frustrated at being unable to help himself."[13]

I also told them he likes to have regular nurses and staff, and appreciates it when people explain what they are doing when in his room.

Roger, our niece Cara, Ruth, Kim, and Sally were all at the meeting, giving me support. There was so much for me to digest that it pushed questions about Brian's infections out of my mind.

Sept 5

S. Diary I arrived to find Brian a little stressed. He was up in his chair for three and a half hours, during which time I was able to take him outside for a while. He seemed to enjoy that. A new nurse was on duty today. I wonder how Brian feels about that after his expressed wish for regular nurses? I am sure that staffing an intensive care unit is not easy.

A blood sample was taken.

Sept 6

S. Diary Stella, Ruth, and I visited today. We found Brian comfortable and a little sleepy. The nurse was having a busy day and had no time to take him outside. We did not stay too late.

Sept 7

S. Diary Kim and Buck did the honours today, choosing a very good time when the patient was up in his chair. Brian showed us more neck movements and put up with the brace for a longer period.

Sept 8

S. Diary Speech therapy started. I have come quite a ways in my lip reading, and it was great to see my husband mouth the words "I love you." How I miss him! I imagine the wondering and guessing will be around for ages.

Sept 9

S. Diary Held Brian's head upright without the brace for ten minutes.

Sept 10

S. Diary Brian's nurse Sonya had him sitting in the wheelchair for almost four hours today. He had his neck brace off under therapist Margot's watchful eye, and he held his head quite steady for what must have been twenty minutes. There is some muscle movement in his shoulders, but nothing in his arms, although Margot is hopeful. She used an electronic stimulator again. Tried to sit him up, but he struggled a bit. Sitting will help strengthen his back and spine. He spelt out more words on the board. What strength he has! I am so proud of him.

Sept 11

S. Diary Brian was really tired after a tough night, and they'd been unable to get the PICC in.[14] Margot and an assistant stopped by to give him more exercises. Someone, not sure who, asked Brian how long he had been there (in Rockyview). His response by means of the communications board was ten minutes! He had a smile on his face, and everyone laughed at his joke. Sonya, his nurse again, was very kind. She keeps a watchful eye over him and is always making sure he is comfortable.

Sept 12

S. Diary Ruth came with me today. She took on the task of redecorating the room, replacing his birthday cards, adding ribbon etc. Brian was doing well, and he followed everything that was going on by moving his head.

* * *

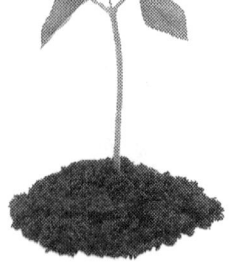

9
Communication Journal Started

On September 13, a communication journal was left by my bed for nurses or visitors to record anything they wished about my progress, achievements, or problems. This was to enable everyone to quickly become updated about my condition. It was nothing more than a hardcover notebook. The idea was suggested by the nursing staff at a recent family meeting. In addition to the continuation of Sylvia's personal diary [S. Diary], excerpts from the communication journal, including the source of each comment, are reproduced here with minor editing.

Sept 13

S. Diary Spent my day off on the golf course with friends Bill and Reta.

Ruth Dad was in the wheelchair around 11AM, and we went outside for half an hour in the afternoon. He was back in bed by 3 PM

Sept 14

S. Diary When I arrived, Brian was trying to move his tongue and left shoulder.

Sylvia Did not take Brian for a walk today since he needed a rest and was comfortable in bed. Earlier, he'd been up in his chair. The doctor, who saw Brian for the first time in three weeks, was very pleased with his progress and told me, "We will take all of the improvements that we can get."

Sept 15

S. Diary Brian had another good nurse today. Ruth and I enjoyed her company and are glad she will be on duty again tomorrow.

Sylvia Sally, Roger, and I saw Brian move his tongue almost to the outside of his mouth. He was very happy about it. He was in his chair from 11AM to 4 PM Had a reasonable day. Lots of smiles.

Ruth Dad didn't go out today. After a few hours, sitting in the chair gets a bit hard on his lower back.

Sept 16

S. Diary Brian was up for about four hours. He asked for a taxi this morning! The doctor wondered if he was trying to be funny. He asked me if Brian had a good sense of humour, to which I replied, "Yes, he certainly has!" Randy calls Brian 'smiler,' which I think makes him feel good. No neck brace today. He is turning his head and holding it in place very well. Later, something seemed to make him angry. Maybe it had to do with using the word board. Perhaps we asked what he believed to be silly questions when we showed him a photograph of a relative and asked who it was.

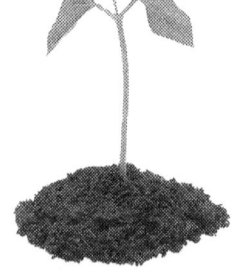

10
Humour Has Its Place

• • •

I do have a sense of humour. In spite of everything I was experiencing, I could often see the funny side of things, although trying to make a joke using an alphabet board rarely, if ever, worked.

In his paper titled Communication and Altered Perceptions Doctor Kopel Burk referred to one of his experiences as a GBS patient on a ventilator and using a speech device. In my opinion, it describes the situation perfectly. Doctor Burk wrote:

> So what happens when you make a joke — especially if one has a habit of laughing at his own jokes? Did someone ask, "How do you laugh on a respirator?" Obviously, one laughs with difficulty. Actually, very few people find anything funny to laugh at while on a respirator.
>
> But since much of what "happens" is internally generated, I often recognized episodes that struck me as funny. What was funny to me then usually was black humor, a bad joke, or a corny pun.
>
> When I tried to make my "funny" comment, it caused something short of pandemonium. Most conversation was intense. The listener worked hard to make sense out of my sounds. Repetition and cadence were critical to understanding anything

> other than a few single words. When I suddenly broke the cadence to insinuate my humor, the listener was confused with a new set of sounds not related to the ongoing conversation.
>
> My wife especially became upset at not being able to understand me. She was my 24-hour-a-day ombudsman and never left me before she was certain that I had no problems, distresses, or anxieties that needed caring for before saying goodnight. The jokes could never be understood with that speech device.
>
> After three or four repetitions, I would pause and rest. I would realize my error in throwing such a monkey wrench into my conversation and I would say, "I'm only making a joke." Such an admission only brought more confusion and anxiety — I had again changed the words and the cadence.
>
> By now I would be exhausted. Once or twice I rolled my eyes in despair, thinking, "How can I be so stupid by trying to be funny under these circumstances?" That eye rolling gesture would only increase my wife's anxiety, and she would plead with me, "Don't be impatient. I can't understand you, but I will stay here all night until I do." I would be filled with guilt to have caused her so much distress.[15]

Speaking is an ability most people take for granted. Unless you have been there, you cannot understand the frustration of not being able to communicate.

Back to the journals and news from overseas:

Sept 16
Sylvia Kath, Jim, and family phoned from England to say hi to Brian. He got up in his chair. The headrest seems better. There had been a problem, but one of the occupational therapists was able to fix it.

Sept 17

S. Diary There aren't enough people available to take Brian outside. He was very proud to show off his shoulder movement.

Sylvia Brian was up for about three hours, but was pretty sleepy for much of the day.

Ruth Dad is very definitely moving his right shoulder up and down. It's good to see, and he is aware of the sensation.

Sept 18

S. Diary Brian was up in his chair for four hours, but was feeling very tired. Lynn Moore, his nurse, was good with him.

Sept 19

Ruth Dad seemed to not be hearing us very well today. Lynn, his nurse again, also commented on it.

S. Diary We are finding it difficult to understand his needs. I am also concerned that he is losing weight.

Sept 20

Sally Dad seemed very tired today, and his eye looked irritated. Later, he appeared to be moving his shoulder and seemed happy with himself.

5:20 PM

Ruth Dad appears to be moving his left shoulder while lying in bed. He's very determined. It looks like he's trying to roll his left side up off the bed.

Sept 21

Sylvia Brian was up in the chair again. The social worker, Yvonne, asked if he would be interested in a visit from a gentleman who had also had Guillain-Barré Syndrome. Brian's response was no, but we'll try again another day. No changes so far today, though his eye seems a little better. I only shaved half his face-need to finish his other side when he's turned over. Lynn noticed a rash around his eyebrows and thinks that, perhaps, he could use a little cream.

S. Diary For some reason Brian was not enthusiastic about his therapy today. All he wanted was his bed. Once again he did not go outside.

Sept 22
Sylvia Brian was up in the chair today, and he is looking better. He's moving both shoulders, has good colour, and smiled a lot. I showed him photos of the garden and a sunflower, which had grown from birdseed. He seemed to be trying to make noises in the back of his throat-I hope we were not dreaming it. Ruth and Sally to visit later.

Ruth Dad communicated to me he was experiencing odd sensations in his head.

Sept 23
Sylvia Brian was very tired today. He wanted to take the plaster off his hand after blood was taken. He could feel it pulling on his hairs, but left it alone. He was up from noon to 3:30 PM I will take him outside if there is someone available to help. The tracheotomy site is weeping, but I told him not to worry about it. It happens quite often. It's a lovely day, and the fall colours are beautiful.

S. Diary The doctor is pleased with Brian's progress and hopes I am taking care of myself. Brian is really working hard to move his right shoulder.

Sept 24

Sylvia Brian was up for four and a half hours and is moving the shoulder quite well. He looks better today and is smiling. His tongue is improving. He loves to show us how he is doing. He asked me not to worry and insisted that it was all right to leave him. My ability to lip read is sometimes better than at other times.

Sept 25

Sylvia Had a great day. Brian was very pleased to see us.

Sept 26

Sylvia Kim, Ruth, and I are here today. Brian is up in his chair, using facial muscles to smile, and moving his neck really well. He wanted his hands exercised.

Ruth Dad hasn't been out for the last few days.

S. Diary Brian's chest appeared to be moving. I hope I am right on this.

Sept 27

Ruth Dad is doing well-we went outside in 22 degrees Centigrade weather.

Sept 28

Sylvia Brian was fairly tired today, but doing okay. They tried some speech therapy. He was up in the chair from 12 – 3 PM The nurses are encouraging him to close his lips and try to blow out. This will help muscles and speech. Pam recommended doing it once or twice. He seems to want to.

Ruth   Ruth in to visit. Goodbye for now — I'm off to China.

S. Diary   Brian was pleased to see us, but didn't particularly want to 'talk'. He doesn't seem stressed about Ruth being out of the country, but I'm sure he will miss her. Me too. I need her strength. I feel I have been relying on her, Kim, and Sally a lot. Thank you all.

Sept 29
Sylvia   Brian was very sleepy all afternoon. He sometimes gets his days and nights mixed up. I've been trying to keep him awake with the TV, but it's not helping. Sleep is his cure. He was in the chair from noon to 3:30 PM

Sept 30
Margot (PT)   Brian moved his right knee at 11:20 AM! It wasn't much of a movement, but four of us saw it.

Sylvia   Thumb moving too.

Sonya   Would it be possible to bring some clothing for Brian — perhaps sweatpants and maybe some short-sleeved shirts so that we can get him dressed when he gets up?

S. Diary   What a day! I arrived to visit Brian and was met by a very excited Yvonne. "Great news!" she said. Brian had moved his knee and thumb! Everyone is so supportive and happy for us, and he was thrilled to be showing everyone what he could do. Way to go! Please keep it up.

Oct 1

Sylvia Family meeting set for today has had to be postponed to October 20.

S. Diary Pam was his nurse today. According to the doctor, Brian still has a bacterial infection, although not a serious one, and his white blood count is high. Fortunately, they don't see a need for drugs.

Oct 2

Sylvia Better day. Brian is smiling a lot, especially when we mentioned he could have a spot of J&B Scotch from a spoon.

S. Diary The doctor told me that Brian will be able to have proper food when his voice returns. That will be great, as we need to start building up his weight.

Oct 3

Sylvia Brian was up in the wheelchair from 10 AM to 2:30 PM I visited with Sally. When he was ready to go back to bed, he was able to tell us so by using his eyes and neck. I read Ruth's news to him.

S. Diary When the patient got back in bed, nurse Teresa made him very comfortable. Sally, who is getting pretty good at lip-reading, saw that he needed the blanket moved off his hands. Although it was only a sheet, it felt heavy to him. He must be feeling something.

Oct 4

Roger There was slight movement in his left hand and also in the right knee. The J&B arrived today and was placed in the cupboard.

Oct 5

Sylvia Brian's nurse took him out for a walk around the back of the hospital. She picked up some autumn leaves for him. For the first time, he asked for a bedpan. The staff is so excited for us. He got up at 11 AM

Oct 6

S. Diary Sheila, my sister-in-law, who had just flown over from England, Roger and myself, found Brian having a good day, moving his head and shoulders really well, and looking so good. Pam was his nurse again, and with help, we got Brian up in his chair for a twenty-minute walk with Helen and Earl. He really enjoyed it. It was a beautiful day, and the autumn colours were spectacular-the best I have seen since we arrived in Alberta over thirty years ago. Everyone is very pleased that Brian is making such good progress.

Oct 7

Sally Dad was up earlier today. He exercised strenuously and is moving his knee and hand a little, also his shoulders. He appears to feel good. He's tired, but then fatigue is another symptom of GBS, right?

Oct 8

Sylvia Sheila and I were greeted with lovely smiles. We brought him a Nottingham Forest tee shirt, and he looked so surprised. Everyone on the team signed it and enclosed a get-well message.[16]

The on-duty nurse suggested we provide tee shirts and boxer shorts for Brian. I took him out for a half-hour walk.

S. Diary Another beautiful autumn day. Brian was very tired after his walk, but he was moving his shoulders and deep breathing well.

Oct 9
Margot Brian moved his left knee into extension by using his hamstrings. It took a lot of help, but he did it. Nothing yet on the right, but I noticed a flicker in his triceps on both sides. I haven't seen his left hand or fingers move yet.

S. Diary Sheila and I were greeted with Margot's news of Brian's progress. After his walk, he was very tired and, as soon as he was transferred back to bed, he fell into a comfortable sleep. Later, he appeared to be experiencing breathing problems. Melissa checked everything out, suctioned him, and he became more restful. He is doing a lot of exercises now, including deep breathing. He must take it easy.

Oct 10
S. Diary Brian was very tired, but comfortable and happy to see Sally, Sheila, and me. Hopefully, he will soon be able to talk to us. All in all, he is doing well. We are so proud of him. Pam and another nurse were looking after him today.

Oct 11
S. Diary Kim and Buck took me to visit, and we found Brian up in his chair under Pam's watchful eye. He was very happy to see us. I am still finding it hard to lip-read.

Oct 12
Sally Dad had lots of company today. Had great smiles for all and wanted us to feel his hands for movement.

··· *A First Step* ···

S. Diary Brian is starting to put some weight back on his face. They are now dressing him each day, which is good for him. Sally was really excited to give me this news. It made her day. Pam was again looking after him.

Oct 13
Sylvia Brian was up from 10 AM to 3:30 PM Roger and Sheila visited with me.

S. Diary Nurse Lynn and Randy were doing the honours today. Brian told Sally he was impatient to start getting around. That's a good sign. I am still struggling with lip-reading and may get five out of ten words! He puckered his lips to give me a kiss. His arms were feeling something, as he indicated the blood pressure recorder band was hurting and asked that it be taken off. Another good sign.

Oct 14
Margot Brian used his shoulder internal rotators today, as well as his triceps. In sitting at the edge of the bed, he was able to bend forward and then straighten up four times! Great progress.

Oct 15
Sylvia Michael came in and cut Brian's hair-it looks great. Roger phoned, and Sheila and I visited in the afternoon. Brian was back in bed and slept most of our visit. Margot is pleased with progress.

S. Diary My brother Colin passed away today after a long struggle with cancer. I thought it best to not pass the sad news on to Brian quite yet. I talked to Pam about it, and she suggested I let them know if and when I decided to tell him so they could keep an eye on him. Speech therapy is to start next week. Brian feels uncomfortable with the cuff in his throat, but Pam thinks he will get used to it. She also gave me the good news that Brian is holding his weight.

Oct 16

S. Diary Sheila, Sally, and I visited and found Brian having a reasonably good day, but later there was a bit of a panic when he had trouble breathing because of the tracheotomy and fluid in his throat. After being suctioned, he settled down. I feel so sad for him. Need to let him know. Sally is marvellous. She is very patient and helps Brian with his exercises.

* * *

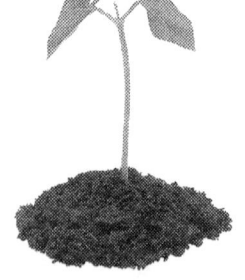

11
Learning to Talk Again

...

Being unable to talk is something none of us can be prepared for. Prior to succumbing to Guillain-Barré Syndrome four months ago, I certainly never gave the possibility a moment's thought. Add to that the inability to write messages, and you are all of a sudden in a very different world.

I was thrilled at the prospect of speaking again. It took me some time to call the valve I was to use by its proper name, which I believe was "Passez- Muir," but no matter. Using it was more important than naming it correctly. It is hard to describe the quiet elation I felt. It was a wonderful feeling to know I could communicate with my wife and other visitors and could talk to my nurses and therapists.

I liked to imagine I was able to convince my doctors that my therapy must not stop until I was as fit as a forty-five year old. Although I am a senior, that was the age I felt like when I succumbed to GBS They were not, I argued, to assume that because of the age on my birth certificate, they could leave me at a lower level of fitness.

And, now, back to the journals:

Oct 17
Unknown Brian had a special valve put on his tracheotomy, which allowed him to speak several words. He did this while sitting up in the chair for about five minutes.

S. Diary	When Sheila and I arrived, Brian had the valve in and said, "I love you, Sylv." What a feeling to hear that! Tears flowed freely. I was on cloud nine.
Unkown	Later he said "Yes" without the special tube in his tracheotomy and asked for the nurse! He was very tired afterwards, but was delighted with himself, as was everyone on ward.

Oct 18

Kim	Brian asked for the special valve to be put in the tracheotomy today. He wanted to talk to Roger, Stella, Mom, and me. His words are quite clear. He said that he has to get used to the new valve.
S. Diary	It is very touching to see Brian's progress. Even the nurses and other staff members are excited about it and the strength he is showing.

Oct 19

Margot	Where is Brian's blue hat with the pointer?[17]
Unknown	The speech valve was in for seventeen minutes. Brian is starting to worry about the expense of being here! I reassured him he would be taken care of by Alberta Health and Blue Cross. Afterwards he seemed more relaxed.
S. Diary	This was a really down day for me. It was my brother Colin's funeral. Nephew Ian phoned from England to describe the service and keep us in touch.

Oct 20

Unknown	The family conference went well. Brian was unable to join us, but perhaps at the next one in December he will be up for it. Today was a better day.

Brian is making progress with his speech and is trying to shape his mouth better. He was on the voice valve for half an hour. I think he needs to go slower. He is feeling pain in the back of his shoulder, which the doctor feels is a sign that his muscles are returning. He was very restless for some time today, and we are keeping eye on him. He needs to sleep, but is always 'chewing away.'

S. Diary Brian performed on the voice valve for Stacy, the respiratory therapist, and she was delighted, even though he was rushing it and making her laugh. He ended up laughing, too. We are still being told that it is going to be a long haul, and it scares me. It must be especially hard for Brian, but as Roger says, he's determined to win.

Oct 21

S. Diary Brian had a stressful day and was feeling pain in the shoulder blade area. Ark and Earl moved him a few times, which helped. He asked for a deep suction. Earlier, he'd been up in his chair for five hours. The speech therapist had him try to mouth different words, using a mirror so he could see himself.

Oct 22

S. Diary Brian has been having some very stressful days and nights, and the doctor is concerned. After a really thorough examination, he thinks Brian may have another urinary tract infection. His lungs appear to be clear. He slept a lot of the time we were there, although Lynn was able to sit him up in his chair for a couple of hours. His neck is much stronger now, and his head did not slip off the headrest. It was good to see. We massaged his shoulders, which he really enjoyed. Roger did one side; I did the other.

Oct 23
Margot Brian demonstrated left shoulder abduction (lifting an elbow out to his side), and he rolled his arms inward so his palm rolled onto the mattress. That's called pronation of the forearm. Yee-haw!

S. Diary It was a beautiful sunny day, and a better day all around for Brian. Lynn was his nurse again.

Oct 24
S. Diary Brian tried to take his Scotch from small cup-we almost poured it into him in tiny drops!! He didn't want swabs. He was much brighter today. I massaged his shoulders again.

Brian's day started out better, but later he experienced what we thought was a panic attack. He had a stressful sensation around his chest and felt trapped. After a deep suction, he soon recovered. He is trying to talk without the valve in and still finding it very hard. Was only up in his wheelchair for two hours, but as I write this, he is feeling better.

Oct 25
S. Diary Sheila left for England this evening. Sally drove her to the airport. Earlier, Sally had entertained us for Sheila's last day. Roger and our niece Cara visited the hospital to give me a day off. It worked out well, since Ruth phoned from Beijing. She sounded happy and was so pleased about Brian's progress.

Oct 26
Sally Roger and Stella stopped in. Dad went outside yes-

terday and today was off the ventilator and breathing on his own for twenty minutes. WOW!

S. Diary   This was a good day. After lunch with Sally, we went to see Brian. Flo, Earl, and Kelly were on duty. Flo explained they were taking Brian off the ventilator for a few minutes to see how he coped with it. He did well, displaying no panic or stress. Another step forward, and I was so pleased that we were there to witness it. The speech therapist was around and explained they were trying to have Brian use his tongue a little more to help with talking. Flo asked him to slow down and spell words.

Oct 27

S. Diary   I think they tired him out today. He had two twenty-minute sessions off the ventilator, breathing on his own and showing no signs of stress. Good for him. Spoke to Yvonne and said I hoped they were not pushing him too fast. She thought not and explained they really want him off the ventilator soon, as it is not good for him to be on it for so long. I needed a good cry. Joan and Carrie (respiratory therapist) were on duty.

Oct 28

Unknown   Ruth phoned Brian from China! We talked to Mark. Snow showers here. Brian seems peaceful today.

S. Diary   Joan Fulton and Carrie were on duty. Brian was excited and so happy to tell me he had talked to Ruth and Mark. The nurse had held the phone to his ear. It was a wonderful tonic, and I think it gave him peace of mind. "What great children we have," I remarked, and Brian, nodded and said, "Yes, don't we." Otherwise, it was a very quiet day. He is breathing on his own for twenty minutes four times a day now and seems very comfortable with it. Meri came in to give him further speech training and worked on using the tongue more.

Oct 29

S. Diary Brian is off the ventilator and breathing on his own for longer each day-half an hour today. Meri was in with the word list to help him practice, but he was too sleepy.

Pam and Earl did the honours today. In spite of being in such good hands, Brian was very weak and made a lot of uncomfortable faces. He had another deep suction. The results from the blood tests aren't in yet.

Oct 30

S. Diary Today Sally and I went to Brian's office to pick up his accumulated mail and some of his belongings. We saw most of the people he used to work with. I think it drained us all. I am so glad Brian was sleeping a lot today. It made it easier to handle.

Nov 1

S. Diary So many visitors today, including Ruth, back from her visit to China. Sally picked her up at the airport and brought her right to the hospital. Brian was excited to see her. Later he complained of discomfort in his shoulders, arms, and hips. Perhaps this is a sign his muscles are regaining strength. The nurse started to cut his fingernails, but it was hurting so much, she only finished one hand. He talked to us for about twenty minutes before we left.

Ruth Dad is asking to be moved a little more frequently.

··· *Learning to Talk Again* ···

He feels the pillows keep him in one position and unable to move if he gets cramped or uncomfortable.

Nov 2

Meri I saw Brian for a session of speech therapy at 12:30 today. He was more alert and responsive and better able to exaggerate his lip and tongue movements. Good session. We reviewed some of the word lists I'd given Sylvia last week.

S. Diary Brian was feeling good when I arrived, although his bottom and hips were a little sore. He was certainly getting lots of attention. Respiratory therapist, Darryl, and therapists Meri and Margot all spent time with him. He is being given more fluid; his heart rate was good, and his blood pressure normal. I had to scratch his nose again! Meri was pleased with his speech.

Nov 3

Margot Brian sat at the edge of the bed unsupported. He held himself up for about twenty seconds. Excellent progress! By the way, there are two physical therapy students here from McMaster University for six weeks who will be assisting me with Brian. With the three of us, I hope we can accomplish some dynamic things.

Pam Brian rubbed his lips together after I had put Vaseline on them. He spoke to me for about an hour. Great day!

S. Diary Pam Barnie and Helen Thornhill were looking after the patient today. He had a good day and was on the voice valve for an hour and a half. His bottom was sore from sitting in the chair for so long.

··· A First Step ···

He refused aspirin for pain, saying he did not need drugs. I was lip reading well and left feeling more relaxed. Sandra will be his night nurse, so he is in good hands.

Nov 4

S. Diary   We celebrated my birthday in Brian's room. He had his days mixed up and thought it was tomorrow. He is feeling frustrated and is ready to move on. He asked me to cancel the arrangements for him to leave on Saturday! Don't know where he got that, as it was the first I or anyone else had heard about it. He now knows that Saturday would be too soon and has decided to stay longer! He worries about nights, as nobody bothers about him. We may be in for a rough time, since he is getting a little short tempered. I left him sleeping. Hope he has a comfortable night.

Nov 5

S. Diary   The doctor on duty told me he was pleased with Brian's progress. Everyone, including Brian's nurse Peggy, was running hard. No one had time for a chat. When Brian needed to sleep, I left, feeling good about the doctor's comment.

Nov 6

S. Diary   Brian is content and in good spirits. He worked hard at his exercises.

Nov 7

Pam   Teeth (top dentures) in for ten minutes.

S. Diary   My day off. Sally went to the hospital, and I was happy to get her phone call letting me know Brian had a good day. Pam and Helen were on duty.

Nov 8

Pam   Brian had his teeth in for half an hour and said his mouth felt cold. Tim, the respiratory therapist, thought it was something else returning. Great news.

S, Diary   Pam and Helen are looking after the patient again today. He was chatty and looked good. Got up in his wheelchair for three hours. He thought I looked more like myself, probably because of my new hairstyle and the fact I was not looking so sad.

Nov 9

Ruth   Dad had his first taste of cranberry juice (on a spoon) today. Comment: "Boy, was that good!"

S. Diary   Brian had a great night. Slept from eleven PM until eight this morning and was very peaceful. He looked good. A rehabilitation table has been set up in his room, ready for tomorrow. They will start working to strengthen the muscles in his back and arms. It will be stressful for him, but it is necessary. Pam and Helen were on duty, along with respiratory therapist Tim and one of his colleagues.

Nov 10

Sylvia   A day of firsts! Brian had his first drink of cold water using a straw and Sally had a first hug. He used the arm rack, which is a contraption that allows the arms of the patient to be raised and move in a horizontal plane, free of gravity. He was out of bed from around eleven until three PM Worked his arms on the exercise machine and did well.

S. Diary   This was Brian's first day of serious rehab. He was strapped to the table, then Margot and her two students put him through his first "off-bed" session.

Margot was impressed. He looked so good and is very positive and sure he is on the road to recovery. New nurses today.

Nov 11

Ruth Dad had apple juice, orange jelly, and water today.

S. Diary Another good day for the most part, although things got quite stressful towards the end when Brian had what I would call a 'panic attack'. This causes his heart rate to jump. One of the respiratory therapists and Lynn, his evening nurse, settled him down after suctioning.

Nov 12

Unknown Today Brian enjoyed some tomato soup through a straw and had a little taste of egg custard and more Jell-O. He enjoyed it, along with the cranberry juice and water. The doctor was pleased and suggested we try mashed potatoes or baby food. Margot came in for exercising-eighteen minutes in all. Brian is now using his arms to pull himself up!

S. Diary Pam, Helen, and later Sandra were looking after our patient today. He did not want to stop his exercising, but must not overdo it. He seems to be handling the fluid in his throat better. I tried to tell Brian that after very generously keeping him on full pay for over six months, his employer would be retiring him at year's end. I am not sure he understood fully, but there were lots of nursing staff and a concerned doctor in and out of his room to cheer him on. I think I am more apprehensive than Brian is.

Nov 13

S. Diary Pam and Helen were on duty today. What a team! Brian was a little tired, but managed some soup, yoghurt, and cranberry juice. Did more physio, sitting on the edge of the bed. His doctor looked in and seemed impressed. He knows Brian is a fighter. Left him with an alarm on his pillow. He feels much safer that way. Not a bad day, really.

Nov 14

S. Diary Brian was a little tired, but cheerful and anxious to get started with physio. Later, he had his speech valve in. Mona was his nurse. He had two teaspoons of barley soup and some mashed potatoes with gravy. Requested physio to come in to help with leg and arm exercises.

Nov 15

S. Diary Mona was in charge again today. It was my day off. Roger, Sally and grandchildren Stephen and Sarah visited. When I'm home, I try to relax, but find it hard. I am still scared about the future and wondering if Brian is going to make it all the way.

Nov 16

S. Diary Brian was on his speech valve for three hours and enjoyed talking to visitors, though he was very tired afterwards. Told us one hand felt warm and the other felt cold. The nurse brought him an extra warm blanket. He exercised on the arm equipment for about thirty minutes or so, and both Ruth and I got hugs.

* * *

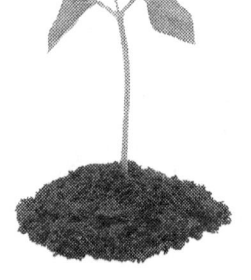

12

Encouragement from an Unexpected Source

Under the banner,

FOREST HELP CANADIAN FAN HIT BY A RARE ILLNESS

the Nottingham Evening Post described the wonderful reaction of the players and staff from the English Premier Division football club, Nottingham Forest, to news of my illness:

> To help his recovery bid, he has been given a boost by players and staff at the City Ground.
> The club was told of his plight and immediately responded by sending him a signed Forest Shirt and a postcard of the City Ground, which are now next to his hospital bed in Calgary.
> And Mr. Langton's younger brother Roger, who also lives in Canada, has been taping Forest videos to show him in hospital.
> Mr. Langton's cousin, Janet .... said; "He was always very fit and healthy. It's terrible to think of him lying in hospital in this condition. It's a very nice gesture of Forest to help him out in this way. He is aware of what is going on around him and this will help him as he battles the illness.[18]

··· *A First Step* ···

Back to the Communication Journal, and Sylvia's dairy:

Nov 17

Dana Brian is having a swallowing test-Meri to be here around 1:15.

Sylvia Brian passed all of the tests and is now able to have juice from a straw.

S. Diary Dana was looking after Brian today. For the swallowing test, he ate half a cup of yoghurt containing blue dye, and he passed with flying colours. When they suctioned him later, there was no trace of the dye. In spite of passing this hurdle, he still could not drink a proper glass of water, and that upset him. He had the speech valve in and talked for a while. Stacy was his respiratory therapist.

Nov 18

S. Diary Again, Brian was in Dana's care. Meri tested him to see if he could handle swallowing clear liquids. So far so good-the first suction recovered no dyed water, and afterwards he looked more comfortable. It was a tiring day for him. They keep him very active, and Margot admitted he had been worked hard at physio. The doctor was impressed with his attitude and fight, but again expressed worry about me.

Nov 19

Unknown Brian moved his knee by himself and had a small movement of the elbow. He read a little today, too, though we had to turn the pages! Very exciting.

Nov 20

S. Diary Arrived at the hospital to find Brian standing! It required the help of four people, but will send

… Encouragement from an Unexpected Source …

his legs the message that they have to work again. Melissa was the duty nurse. Brian was on his voice valve from 9:00 AM to 9:00 PM Twelve whole hours! I wish his ventilator did not beep so often, but apparently it is due to air leaks.[19]

Nov 21

Unknown Again today, Brian's voice valve was in for a long time. The children were happy Grandpa could talk and say 'Happy Birthday' to Kim. It was a good day.

S. Diary We celebrated Kim's birthday in Brian's room. The girls and I contributed cakes, finger bites, cheese biscuits, and fruit. Melissa and the other nurses were invited to join the party.

Nov 22

Ruth Dad watched the Grey Cup today.

S. Diary They are seeing how it goes without a catheter today. Nancy and Stacy (his nurse and respiratory therapist) worked hard with him. The speech valve was in nearly all day so it was easier to chat.

Nov 23

Sally Ruth and I came in today-Mum's day off. Dad had trouble catching his breath this morning. The x-ray showed a mucus plug in the left lung.

S. Diary Brian was in Nancy's good hands again today. He required deep suctioning.

Nov 24

S. Diary Brian sent me flowers! What a surprise and wonderful tonic! He had obviously arranged the surprise delivery with the girls' help. He had a good

··· A First Step ···

day, too, and was glad to tell me the x-rays were clear. He did really well with his arm exercises, is looking quite fit, and holding his weight.

Nov 25

S. Diary It was a great day. Brian raised his left arm by himself and did more with his right arm than he has been. They are not planning to transfer him out of Intensive Care yet, though, because of his continuing need for assisted breathing. I helped to feed him Sally's homemade soup, fruit jelly, and cherry yoghurt. Talked to the social worker, Yvonne, and she was surprised at his progress, in spite of the news from the doctor.

Nov 26

S. Diary Another good day with Flo and Earl looking after the patient. The doctor talked to Brian about a trach cork, which he wants him to try six times a day for about ten to fifteen minutes at a stretch. He didn't think Brian would be stressed, and the respiratory therapists, including Kelly, will monitor him very carefully.[20]

Nov 27

S. Diary Brian had the same nursing team as he did yesterday. Flo soaked his feet and cut his nails. I took care of his hands. Brian was happy to show me how much he can move his left arm and shoulder now. Respiratory therapists were Kelly and another young assistant.

Nov 28

S. Diary Brian was up in his chair when I arrived. His bottom was sore from sitting, and his feet were very tender and swollen. He didn't complain, though, and otherwise looked surprisingly comfortable.

Encouragement from an Unexpected Source

Nov 29

S. Diary   Kim and I visited and found Brian somewhat tired, but comfortable. I think he enjoys the quiet of Saturdays and Sundays.

Nov 30

S. Diary   Beulah was on duty for the third day. I had lunch with our patient. A neurology specialist visited him regarding pain and tingling sensations in his feet. Could this be GBS returning? Unbeknownst to us, he was prescribed a painkiller twelve days ago. Today Brian said he preferred to bear the pain and promised that if it got too much for him, he would ask for the medication.

Dec 1

S. Diary   Had a good visit and watched Brian do a few sit-ups on the edge of his bed. No records were broken, and he found it a little uncomfortable due to badly fitting underwear, but still it is progress. He also needs wider fitting shoes and socks. Today and tomorrow Pam will be keeping an eye on him, ably assisted by Helen.

Dec 3

S. Diary   Another good day. Brian said he just wanted to look at me! Supported from behind by the physiotherapist Donna, he held himself up for a few minutes and then tried to move from side to side. Beulah was doing the honours.

* * *

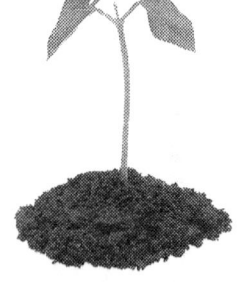

13
Some Reflections on Life in Intensive Care

It often takes something like this to make one fully appreciate the wonder of life, and the miracle that is man.
—Brian Langton

What were some of my later recollections of life in the intensive care ward? One thing that comes readily to mind was the never-ending supply of warm blankets, which felt like they came straight from the oven. They were so welcome and soothing.

I recall the longest and possibly the most uncomfortable time of each day being early morning around the shift change. I could not wait to learn who my nurse was to be and was always anxious for him or her to come in and attend to whatever discomfort had awakened me. Sometimes it was an itchy nose or ear, sometimes the fact that my back was uncomfortably placed on the crease, which felt like a hinge running side to side across the centre of my airbed.

I could hear the new staff coming in and taking reports from the outgoing night staff, though some mornings it seemed to me that they were having a party. At other times, I would imagine they were frequenting a cafeteria in place of the nursing station. I could see it very vividly in my mind's eye. There were colourful umbrellas at each table, and the nursing staff would all be enjoying coffee and relaxing. I would lie in bed trying to will someone to come into my room.

A First Step

There were very few negatives, though; and those that existed, such as the lack of attention during shift changes, were for the most part, unavoidable.

The positives were many. I felt very fortunate for the tremendous amount of attention I received through much of the day. The nurses and aides were attentive and, when time permitted, we enjoyed some good conversations, often with lots of humour thrown in. Once I could talk, I used to give one of the respiratory therapists as hard a time as she gave me.

"Oh no! Not you again," I would joke as she entered the room.

Her reply would be something like, "Well, I'm sorry, but no one else was willing to come." Even when I was in dire need of suctioning, it was great to have some fun at the same time.

I often reflected on my good fortune to have such a pleasant view from my window. There was a park with beautiful trees, and I could see the footpaths around Glenmore Reservoir, although the trees hid the reservoir itself from my view. More often than not, the blue Alberta sky was very much in evidence, providing a perfect backdrop. One of my doctors commented that it was, perhaps, the best view from any intensive care room in the country. I could see joggers, people walking their dogs, and those who were out for a leisurely walk. I was quite sure that few, if any, of them considered just how lucky they were to be able to get around on their own steam. Unlike me, lying virtually paralysed in a hospital bed, they could make forward progress automatically, without thinking. They did not have to make a decision to raise a foot, concentrate on swinging it forward and landing it firmly heel first, and then repeat it all with the other foot. They just did it. I was like them before my illness struck. By this time, however, I knew that I was going to have to learn all over again to walk and talk and eat and do all the other things people take for granted. It often takes something like this to make one fully appreciate the wonder of life and the miracle that is man.

Someone, such as my chest physiotherapist, would often disturb these thoughtful moments. I enjoyed her visits. In spite of the chest pummelling I had to endure, it was always good to have the company. Then there were the welcome visits from family and friends.

Some Reflections on Life in Intensive Care

I have never ceased to be amazed and gratified at the love, endurance, and extreme patience shown by my wife. How truly lucky I was.

In her journal, Sylvia next describes another typical day, but one with a very different, though welcome, visitor:

Dec 4

S. Diary Ruth and I arrived in the middle of a physiotherapy session. Brian was working his arms hard, doing a great job, and did not look stressed. The doctor is happy with the way he is clearing fluid from his lungs. He is looking fit and well, eating better, and holding his weight. The nurses have suggested a night out for Brian to see the Christmas lights. This will be doable so long as a nurse and respiratory technician are available, and it would be a wonderful change for Brian. Respiratory therapist Carrie brought in her eleven-week-old puppy, a cute Labrador. Brian was thrilled.

Dec 5

S. Diary Sally visited today while I got involved with Christmas cooking at home to cheer myself up. Pam and Helen were looking after him, doing their excellent work.

Dec 6

S. Diary Appearing to be in good spirits, Brian was up in his chair for a couple of hours, but needed to go back to bed earlier than Pam wished. She explained that for his own good, he must be out of bed for a longer period. She also had him on the trach cradle for a while.[21] It was not too busy. Kim and Robert were with me and helped to decorate the room for Christmas. Robert put up a poster he made.

Dec 7

S. Diary   Brian complained of a dry throat and has a canker sore in his mouth. I hope it is not an infection. Otherwise, he is doing well. Moved his knee and really wanted us to work him hard and move him around. Pam is on again, with Ark taking over later. Tim was the respiratory therapist helping Brian today.

Dec 8

S. Diary   Brian was doing exercises when I arrived. He has resumed taking vitamin C, which should help his mouth and throat. Stacy — never a dull moment for Brian when she is around — was his respiratory therapist. I brought in some cheese straws I baked and left some for Beulah, his night nurse. Brian seemed quite content.

Dec 9

S. Diary   Brian had a bad day. He had fluid in his left lung and was given a deep suction, which removed a lot of angry-looking fluid. I am worried about pneumonia, although the doctor isn't, at least not yet. They are keeping a close eye on him, and he is getting regular attention from the respiratory therapists. He was on the ventilator all day. Lip reading again was quite difficult. I am able to read most of his words, but it will be nice to get back to normal and start making progress again. Lynn phoned me at home later in the evening to let me know Brian said he was feeling better and that it was not pneumonia. That was so good to know.

Dec 10

S. Diary   A family conference today, and this time Brian was included. He thanked everyone for being there with special appreciation to his daughters, his brother, and me and for what we are doing for him. He had most of the team in tears. He mentioned some diet preferences and said he was still finding it hard to swallow, but, otherwise, was feeling better. The doctor said he would be pushed harder at rehabilitation and that, so far, all the therapists were pleased with him.[22]

Later, Pam and Helen, and RT Stacy watched as we added to the Christmas decorations.[23]

Meanwhile, Brian was back on the trach cradle, although he is still a little hoarse. At his own request, he is no longer taking pain or sleeping meds. He has managed to convince the doctor he does not need them.

Dec 11

S. Diary Ruth and I had supper with Brian, and he really enjoyed it. He was not too patient with one of the respiratory therapists, and I felt sorry for her. The nursing staff is trying so very hard to help, but he seems to be trying to control them and the care he is receiving. I suppose it represents a desire to be back in control of his life in general. His moods and attitude are different with them, but he is all right with me. In spite of it, he is coping well.

Dec 12

S. Diary A much better day. Brian was much more relaxed. Nurse Donna, supported by a respiratory therapist, was looking after him. One of the physiotherapists put him through his paces with close to one and a half hours of exercises. It tired him out, but he did more later.

··· *A First Step* ···

Dec 13
S. Diary   I had my day off to do some Christmas baking. Ruth and Sally visited their Dad.

Dec 14
Ruth   Dad reported a flicker of movement at the top of his right hand.

Dec 15
S. Diary   Brian was quite alert and very bossy with the nurses! He still has fluid on the left lung, and they are keeping an eye on it.

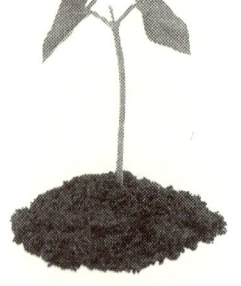

14
Approaching Yuletide

* * *

A hospital was not the best place to be at Christmas, but then neither was being on guard duty in Aldershot, United Kingdom, as I was on a bitterly cold Christmas Day many years ago. One does not always know what destiny has in store. I was, however, fortunate. The nursing staff and my family were doing what they could to give me the best Christmas possible. The nurses arranged for me to see the Christmas lights in downtown Calgary, which involved procuring transportation, a volunteer nurse, a respiratory technician, and a driver. I was humbled and very grateful for their wonderful gesture.

The trip went almost as planned. As we got under way, I realized that I hadn't worn a neck brace, and my neck muscles were not nearly as strong as I had imaged. I felt unable to hold my head stable when we hit even the slightest bump in the road. This being December, there were patches of ice and the inevitable potholes. Happily for me, my very experienced respiratory therapist took matters literally into his own hands and held onto my head for a good part of the evening. He also administered just enough oxygen to keep me comfortable.[24]

We were supposed to go straight downtown, but then someone had the bright idea to run out to Cochrane, a small town West of Calgary, where there was a spectacular Christmas lighting display at the Western Heritage Centre. No objections were raised, so that is where we headed. I saw the funny side of this. Here I was, out on the town for the first time in six months, and at the first chance

··· *A First Step* ···

I choose to leave town and hit the highway. On a more serious note, I wondered what my chances would be if we were to become stuck in the snow somewhere and I ran out of oxygen.

I need not have worried, we had an excellent driver.

The lighting display was worth the trip. After viewing it from several angles, we made our way back to the city. We didn't go directly back to the hospital, but drove to see some of the lights in town. It was a truly wonderful evening, made possible by some very caring and unselfish people.

Sylvia describes the outing, from her point of view, in her journal:

Dec 16

S. Diary Brian was in good spirits today and being looked after by nurse Loverna. A friend of the family cut his hair. The doctor, who is talking to him more, is delighted with his progress. An outside trip had been arranged for Brian to see the Christmas lights. At about seven thirty that evening Ruth and I accompanied him, his nurse Nancy, and an experienced respiratory therapist, who was charged with holding his head in an upright position.

Nancy wore earrings with tiny flashing coloured lights for the occasion. I understand both the driver and the respiratory therapist volunteered their time so Brian could get out of the hospital for the first time in five or six months. What seemed like a normal ride to us, he described as 'bumpy', and he wasn't able to hold his head steady. Nancy let him have a beer, when he got back to his bed. He was the talk of the ward. Everyone wanted to make sure he was all right.

Dec 17

S. Diary Lynn cared for Brian, and he had a good day. He's moving his arms more, holding his weight, and looking good. He's off the protein drip now and always ready for his meals.

Dec 18

Unknown Brian was breathing with the trach cork in for twenty minutes. He was able to swallow a sip of dyed water, and the suction was clear. He didn't feel so stressed as on a trach cradle. Another step forward to weaning him off the ventilator!

S. Diary Brian felt corking was easier. He could talk normally and is in good spirits. His eyes are really sparkling. Ark was the nurse on duty.

Dec 19

S. Diary Pam was on duty again, with respiratory therapist Tim and his colleague overseeing Brian on the trach cork. Again, he did well. He enjoyed my rubbing his legs and feet and wanted me to resist him pushing with his arms. I could see the arm muscles moving, but nothing in the fingers, although I know there will be movement eventually. At his request, his Vitamin C intake has been increased. It was a cold day-minus 28 degrees Centigrade.

Dec 20

S. Diary My day off. Brian has told me I must not visit if the weather is really bad. It is another cold day.

Dec 21

S. Diary Apart from being on the tilt table, Brian was in bed all day. He said being on his feet felt good. He moved his waist from side to side, and Margot was impressed with the pushing of his arms. Pam was on duty again.

When I arrived home, I received a beautiful bouquet of flowers for Christmas from Brian. Just looking at them will help me through the holidays.

Dec 22

S. Diary   Brian is in good spirits. Again, he worked hard on the tilt table. As he pushed tables away and pulled them back, we could see his muscles working. Nurse Sonya was on duty, with respiratory therapist Carrie. He was back in bed about three PM.

Dec 23

S. Diary   I needed a day to unwind. Had my hair permed and received a beautiful bouquet of flowers from Brian's company.

Dec 24

S. Diary   Christmas Eve-a very sad and difficult day for all of us. Christmas is such an important occasion in our family. I hope it will be over quickly this year. Pam is looking after Brian today.

Dec 25

S. Diary   Sally and Dwayne had me with them to open their Christmas gifts. They gave me a great morning, then it was off to the hospital. We were with Brian from about 2:00. The nurses, so unselfishly on duty this Christmas Day, allowed our daughters to set up a finger food table in his room, along with a miniature wine and sherry bar. Everyone was there-our sons-in- law, our grandchildren, and Roger, too. We opened a few presents.

It was a happy day, given the circumstances, but we all felt drained and it took some effort to be brave and strong. When we started to sing carols, there were more than a few tears. Many of the nurses and respiratory therapists Stacy and Darryl also shared some of the day with us.

Dec 26

S. Diary It was very busy in Intensive Care. Respiratory therapist Darryl was on duty. Brian mentioned that it is just about six months since he was first admitted to Rockyview Emergency and suggested we start to count the days until his homecoming. He is forecasting March. It does me so much good listening to his thoughts and realizing the strength he has to fight. Friends John and Robyn came by, and that made him happy.

Dec 27

S. Diary Roger visited his brother today. It was snowing very hard and was much colder. I am glad Christmas is over and we can now start a new phase.

Dec 28

S. Diary I had a streaming cold and phoned to see how Brian was. His nurse gave me an update and told me he was really fine. I felt bad for not visiting again, but I know he will understand and be glad that I stayed at home.

Dec 29

S. Diary Stayed home again, although I felt a little brighter. Brian was in good hands, though, having Pam and Sandra as his nurses. Sandra arranged for him to telephone me about five PM to say he was feeling fine. He stressed that I should not visit until I felt better.

... A First Step ...

Dec 30
S. Diary   I was still not well. Brian phoned again. It sounded so good to hear his voice.

Dec 31
S. Diary   Happy New Year! I got Brian on his side, and he helped by turning his shoulders. I'll never make an artist! Ha. Ha. (Arleen, N.A.). *Cute 'matchstick men' drawings followed.*

Roger and Stella are visiting in my place today and tomorrow. I feel so helpless with this cold. It is New Year's Eve. Maybe the next year will see things turn around for all of us. Let's hope so.

Jan 1
S. Diary   Happy New Year! Let's be positive and sail into better times. Feeling better, but will not visit until tomorrow, as Brian asked me to take it easy until I am completely well. Better safe than sorry. Our golfing friends Bill and Reta visited him and stayed over two hours.

Jan 2
S. Diary   Not a bad day. It was much warmer and there was a 'Chinook' feeling in the air.[25]

When I arrived, Helen was looking after Brian. He did some 'corking' for about half an hour and was looking so much better. Tim, his respiratory therapist was very pleased with his progress.

Jan 3
S. Diary   Pam and Helen were doing the honours today. They were a little worried about Brian's right lung, as it was somewhat noisy. When the respiratory therapists suctioned him, they could hear crackling. Grandson Robert visited Brian with me. We found

him in a real good mood in spite of the lung problem. He is confident he will be moving around soon and is looking forward to more rehabilitation.

Jan 4

S. Diary   A better day. My cold seems to be going, but I am wearing a mask and scrubbing, just in case. Margot and one of her assistants were working on Brian's rehabilitation program. They had him sit on the edge of the bed without support. He did five pushes forward from the waist, then pushed himself back. He was very proud of himself and did not look at all stressed.

Jan 5

S. Diary   Brian was pleased to see me. He did well with rehab again and impressed Margot with his progress.

Jan 6

S. Diary   Today there was forty-eight minutes of cork cradling; then he was on the tilt table doing exercises, including moving his knees backwards and forwards. It was a great day and the second one for nurses Terrell and Lynn. Brian is looking forward to a walk in Fish Creek Park.[26] We made it a date. He was so positive and feeling better and stronger. The doctor was impressed with his improvement in the last three weeks and commented on how far he has come. Margot thought he had been touched by an angel.

Jan 7

S. Diary   The family meeting slated for two PM was cancelled due to sickness and emergencies in the ICU Brian was comfortable and still talking about coming home. Margot added a note of caution, saying we still had a long way to go, but she was impressed with his progress. He turned himself over in bed, with assistance.

Jan 8
S. Diary Brian was more tired today. As usual, respiratory therapist Stacy tried to make him smile. Nurse Pam told me he had progressed from having acute chronic axonal G.B.S to simply chronic axonal GBS Even though we are out of the acute phase, there is still have a long way to go. Nurse Terrell came on duty in time for a 4:00 meeting we had with the doctor, who wants to set up weekly meetings that include Brian. This will encourage him to set goals for himself. In the meantime, he may have to practice patience, as the staff is quite busy with more seriously ill patients.

Jan 9
S. Diary Nurse Mona was very kind to us. I must have looked sad, as both she and Lynn were worried about me. It has been a long six months. Brian and I discussed the implications of yesterday's meeting. I can't help feeling he is in the way in ICU He can't expect the level of attention he used to get from the staff when he was much sicker. I massaged his legs and helped him bend his knees.

Jan 10
S. Diary My day off. Al visited, and Brian was on the trach cork for six and a half hours. Great progress.

Jan 11
S. Diary Brian was in good spirits when I reached the hospital. Ark was the nurse, supported by nursing aid Randy. Brian enjoyed a good lunch and is get-

ting stronger by the day. Corked for six and a half hours again. (SJ).

Jan 12
S. Diary A great visit today. Flo, Earl, and respiratory therapist Stacy were on. Brian was on the tilt table, encouraged by Margot, Allison, and a new therapist named Jane, who will be taking over from Margot. He had a very hard workout and was raring to go.

Jan 13
Unknown Brian held himself up on the edge of the table for five minutes, moving from side to side. When he put his elbows down on the table, he felt pressure as he pulled himself up, but managed it with a little help! He had a good day. Jane, Allison, and Margot were impressed. He helped Flo to roll him over to use a bedpan and was able to keep stable. Great progress.

S. Diary Brian has been amazed at how well I have handled his illness, how strong I have been, and how I have always been there for him. It is hard sometimes, but I always try to have a cheerful smile whenever I am with him. He had a really good session of physiotherapy today and remarked how good it was to feel his legs under him. He said he felt like he should be able to walk down the hallway, although he knows that to be impossible, at least for now. Thanks to Flo and Earl for caring for him again. What a wonderful job the nursing staff does. Flo, for example, takes care of all those little personal things and makes Brian so comfortable. He did corking for nearly nine hours. Come home soon Brian, and let us start living again.

··· *A First Step* ···

Jan 14

Unknown Brian was impressed by his ability to move with more confidence, and he had a smile on his face!!

S. Diary It appears Brian has a touch of diabetes. Maybe it will go away as he gets better. He had another strong workout on the tilt table, sitting and doing side-to-side pushovers using his elbows for support. Stella was with me and massaged his shoulders for a good fifteen minutes. His nurse was very sweet and nursing aid Earl treats him like a gentleman.

Jan 15

S. Diary Brian on the trach cork now for nine to ten hours a day and gets only five percent help from the ventilator through the night. Today he was interviewed by a doctor from the Foothills Hospital. Apparently he is being considered for admission to their rehabilitation ward, which it seems can offer more suitable rehab, consistent with Brian's needs. The doctor gave him a very thorough examination and told me there would not be one-hundred-percent recovery without more help of the kind Foothills can offer. Brian was okay with it, but concerned that it would involve more travel time for me.

Jan 16

S. Diary Roger, Ruth, and I were pleased for Brian when Pam told us that Foothills Hospital would accept him for rehabilitation. The doctor feels he is able to handle it, and Brian feels ready and is so keen to be on with the program. He made us laugh with his descriptions of the dreams he experienced in his early days in intensive care. He was laughing too, but had been a little worried at the time he was experiencing some of them. He could not remember much of the early days spent at the Foothills, but maybe that is not a bad thing. He is working hard now on coming home.

Jan 17
S. Diary Pam is again looking after Brian and witnessed the start of what was to be his record thirteen and a half hours off the ventilator. He had been challenged by the on-duty doctor to go twelve or thirteen hours.[27]

Jan 18
S. Diary Brian's days are so long, but he is sleeping better and holding his weight. He was a little tired today. Pam and the rest of the staff were extremely busy, as there is a shortage of beds and we seem to be at the peak of the flu season.

Jan 19
S. Diary Brian had a good day, but they put him in a new chair, and he was not comfortable in it. He felt the older chair was more suitable. He also worries about his being transferred to and from the bed in a 'cot'. The nurses handle him more carefully when transferring him manually, but it requires more people. He felt some pain in his feet and his ankles were swollen, but that could have been from the 'cot' transfer.[28]

Jan 20
S. Diary Brian is not experiencing light-headedness or dizziness on the tilt table, which is good. He did a few shoulder pushes at physiotherapy. His shoulders and back are getting much stronger now. He sat up in the original chair for a couple of hours and then

went back to bed. He was off the ventilator for nearly fourteen hours. His feet are less swollen.

Jan 21

S. Diary   Weaning Brian off the ventilator, changing him to a diet of minced foods, and getting him wearing dentures were the main topics at the doctor's meeting with him this morning. It was a tough day for him, trying to cope with all he was told and being concerned about the possibility of a move to another ward. In spite of everything, he still wants to golf. Good for him.

Jan 22

Unknown   Target for corking today is sixteen hours.

Unknown   Brian moved his left toes and knee a few times. He was very excited about it. He sat in the new chair from 3:15 until 5:30 PM and was more comfortable this time. He also went without oxygen for an hour and forty-five minutes and feels better about himself today.

S. Diary   A wonderful day! Brian got more attention from Pam and Flo. He was off oxygen completely for two hours before he realized it. He showed a lot of interest in the hand-held Pulse Oximeter, which was being used to read the percentage of oxygen saturation in his blood. As long as his oxygen saturation was in the 92/93 range, he was very relaxed. I think any reading over 90 is good. His respiratory therapists were Stacy and Christine. He was in another new chair for two and a half hours and found it much more comfortable than the first one they tried. He was moving his knee and both legs better. In general, he was pleased with his progress.

* * *

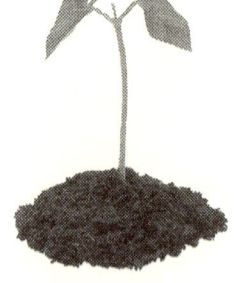

15
Better Days

Just a year ago, Sylvia and I were enjoying a wonderful holiday in Maui, Hawaii. I think it was perhaps the best holiday we have ever had. It mattered little that we had to drive to the airport at four in the morning when the temperature was minus 35° Centigrade. In contrast, as we were on our early morning approach to Kahului, Maui's International Airport, I remember the captain on our Canada 3000 flight announcing that the temperature at our destination was a mere plus 15° Centigrade — 'one awful day in paradise.'

It seemed quite appropriate to receive a post card from one of my respiratory technicians who was holidaying in that wonderful part of the world and complaining of sunscreen in her eyes, seawater up her nose, and surviving a seven hour flight to get there. I could feel the pain she was suffering! In addition to her card, I was surrounded by get-well cards and artwork. The Christmas decorations were gone, but I now had a large chessboard hung on the wall to record the progress of a game I was playing with Mark, who would send me his moves from China.

Now after thoughts of Maui, and China, back to reality in Calgary and much more mundane affairs:

Jan 23
S. Diary Dentures are perhaps going to be a problem. I wonder if the dentist would visit to check them out? Brian was lifting his arms more and trying to move his thumb.

A First Step

Jan 24

Kim   Brian was breathing with the trach cork for twenty-four hours yesterday. Great work! Keep it up; you're well on your way.

Robert & Brian   Well done Grandpa!!

S. Diary   My day off. In the evening I got a surprise phone call from Brian. He had been off the ventilator all night and did not feel too bad. It is wonderful that his lungs are now functioning on their own.

Jan 25

Sylvia   I was told today they will be moving Brian out of ICU to a ward upstairs. I am to meet the new caregivers. He is off the ventilator completely now. Great work, Brian! The patient care manager came in to talk to him. He will know most of the doctors and meet a few new ones.

S. Diary   Great news. Although he still needs to be in isolation, Brian is to be transferred out of Intensive Care to a private room in a medical ward. He is now off the ventilator, and even the equipment has been taken out of his room.[29]

He had a good forty-minute rehab session. We all thought we saw some movement in his left thumb, but it did not repeat, so we have to wait and see.

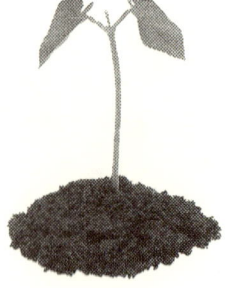

16
Breathing on My Own

After seven months, almost to the day, I was finally free of the ventilator. This was key. If I were to get well again, I had to be able to breath on my own. It was a huge relief and a clear indication that I had reached a vitally important milestone. I surprised myself in not being too apprehensive at having lost this crutch. My lungs were still somewhat compromised, but I could work on that.

Back to the journals and some big changes now I was no longer tied to a ventilator:

Jan 26

S. Diary Pam was on duty when I arrived. The respiratory therapists were Tim and Christine. I went with Brian to rehab. He sat up for fifteen minutes and looked so normal to me. He did pushes side-to-side, backwards, and forwards against pressure. He is very positive. When I suggested he might be coming home by August, he shook his head and said it would be sooner than that.[30]

Jan 27

Sylvia Great day! They moved Brian out of ICU room 9 to 7406, a south-facing private room with a bath. I think everyone who was on duty in the ICU came by to hug him and wish him well.

A First Step

S. Diary A big day for Brian. He was transferred from Intensive Care to a medical ward. It is seven months, almost to the day, that life took a scary turn for us. Now we are in the home stretch, and Brian is very positive and upbeat. Unit 74, his new home away from home, was a little busy, and I think we were both a little unnerved by the move, even though it is a good one. His new nurses were very attentive and quickly helped settle him in. The doctor told us that the trachea and intravenous tubes would be removed very soon.

...

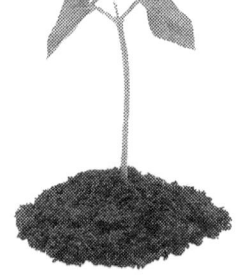

17
Light at the End of the Tunnel

• • •

I recall January 27 very clearly. After almost seven months of dedicated care and exceptional attention, I was very comfortable and secure in Intensive Care and not too enthused when I was advised that my impending transfer would happen within a couple of hours. I had been led to believe there would be at least a twenty-four hour notice, but I guess they needed my bed.

A lot of things were going through my mind, not the least of which was that I was going to miss everyone who had been a part of my daily life in the ICU for so many months. I knew I was leaving a safe haven for something closer to the outside world and that the same level of attention could not be expected. Even though I knew it was the next step on the road to recovery, my feelings were mixed.

I think my biggest fear was that there might not be a respiratory therapist around to suction me if I needed it. I knew I was being somewhat neurotic-that the ward nurses were quite capable of providing a suctioning should one be called for; but the thought worried me just the same. In spite of everything, I was looking forward to the move.

The morning of January 28 dawned to find me settling into my new quarters. On one hand, it was a little troubling to know I was no longer a special case; but on the other, it meant I was getting better, even if only slowly. I was aware that there would not be enough

··· A First Step ···

staff to lift me from bed to chair and it would have to be done by cot every time. That was not very comfortable, but there was really no alternative.

The one common thread was my daily physio and occupational therapy sessions, which were still held in "the basement". That, thankfully, remained unchanged.

I knew I was now on a different part of my journey, and if I were to recover fully, the next months would require a good deal of dedicated effort. I recall thinking that I'd probably experience discomfort and would tire easily, but if that is what it would take, so be it. I made no secret of the fact I was going to beat GBS and would get back to doing everything I had done previously, including playing golf.

Not everyone agreed. In fact I was told many times that my expectations were too high. It had even been suggested that I would never walk again.

I was not a good listener. In fact, my usual reaction was to give the messenger a wry smile, shake my head, and say quite simply, "You are wrong. I intend to golf again."

Although I saw the medical ward I was now in as a transition between Intensive Care and the rehabilitation ward at a different hospital, my rehab had actually had it's origins back in ICU, where the dedicated professionals had started me on the road to recovery.

Another peek at the diary maintained by Sylvia indicates the progress being made, albeit slowly, starting from the second day in my new unit:

Jan 28
S. Diary Brian did sitting exercises under the watchful eyes of his therapists, and then they tried to get him to stand. That was a bit frightening. He had not been able to straighten up for many months. Afterwards, he was in his chair for over two hours.

Jan 29
S. Diary Brian was in his chair for two hours again today, though there was some discomfort in his calf and buttocks. It is a pity he cannot move around himself.

Jan 30
S. Diary   Sally and I both thought we saw Brian's thumb move. It was a great feeling. He did not stay in his chair for long, as he was experiencing some pain in the upper left leg.

Feb 1
S. Diary   The doctor wanted Brian off oxygen for the whole day. Brian is quite happy about this, provided the monitor, which he loves to play with, registers 92 or greater. Anything less and he worries. Up in his chair for two and a half hours, his legs are still feeling tender. Physiotherapy is going well.

Feb 2
S. Diary   A positive day at physio. With a little help, Brian succeeded in pulling himself up, but his bed is a problem. He also seems to be having difficulty with some of the night staff, who seem to know nothing about GBS.[31] He had a bad night off the oxygen. When checked, his 02 reading was only 82/85. He was put back on.

Feb 3
S. Diary   Brian had a good rehab session and appeared to be enjoying it. With the help of four therapists, he stood upright three times and experienced tension only in his thighs and knees. He is forecasting he will be home in eighty-four days. That would be the end of April. We will see!

Feb 4
S. Diary   A busy day. Brian did lots of physio and had a visit from his dentist, who took an impression to enable the relining of Brian's denture. In spite of the dentist being so careful, it was awful for Brian to

hold still and not gag with the mixture in his mouth. Later, when he has his denture back, I am sure he will be glad.

Feb 5

S. Diary   Brian is in good spirits and able to move his knee to get more comfortable when in bed. Great stuff.

Feb 6

S. Diary   Brian was very uncomfortable in the chair today. He's feeling aches and pains in his thighs and lower legs. He was not happy to miss soup today and, on top of everything else, he missed seeing his favourite soccer team, Nottingham Forest of the English Premier Division, on television.

Feb 8

S. Diary   Physio was cancelled for the day, as Brian was complaining of a sore throat after the feeding tube was taken out of his stomach. He was sleepy all afternoon and certainly has a cold. The dentist returned with the dentures, and they appear to be a good fit.

Feb 9

S. Diary   Brian was much brighter and appears to be fighting off his cold. He did light physio; ate his first solid food in over seven months; and was comfortable with his denture.

Feb 11

S. Diary   For the first time Brian expressed anger at having caught the Guillain-Barré Syndrome virus and having his life taken from him for such a long time. It has been hard for us, too, but even though we still have a difficult stretch ahead of us, I feel we have come a long way.

Feb 14

S. Diary   Brian ate good meals today and felt brighter. He made a chess move in the game he is playing with Mark, who is still in China. It creates a lot of interest. Brian came to sit with us in the lounge overlooking the reservoir. It was a beautiful day.

Feb 15

S. Diary   Getting things ready for Brian's pending transfer to the Foothills Hospital. His left leg gave him some discomfort while he was in his chair.

Feb 16

S. Diary   Although it was another big day for Brian on his road to recovery, it was quite unsettling for him and for us! He was transferred to the rehabilitation ward at the Foothills, which meant saying goodbye to so many people who have done so much for him. Many who were off duty came in especially to see him, including nurse Pam, therapists Jane, Allison, Meri, and several other respiratory therapists I did not know. It was all very touching. The transfer went well, and the reception at Foothills was very pleasant. I met Norma, who will be one of Brian's nurses, and Brenda, who will be his physiotherapist.

* * *

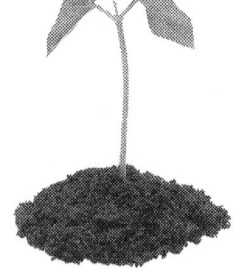

18
Another Big Step Forward

This, then, was the final lap. I was now in the rehabilitation ward at Foothills Hospital, the move that preceded my discharge from hospitals. When I first arrived, I did not feel entirely ready for the full rehabilitation program, but it had to be started sometime.

Most of the concerns and fears I experienced in the early days of my illness were still with me. The fear of being left alone and unable to move or communicate, for example, was paramount. Granted, I could now speak and even call out (assuming help was within hailing distance, which I found to be rarely the case); but my ability to move was still very limited, and being unable to use my arms and hands, I could do little to help myself.

I believe it was at this time that I began to experience itching, chiefly on my face and around my ears. Perhaps it had something to do with the nerves coming back to life in those areas. Ironically, this was also the time when there were few people available to respond to my calls for help. The night staff most certainly did not appreciate it when I hit the call button just to have my nose scratched, and yet the need was often most desperate. I soon learned to call for some other reason and, as a supposed afterthought, ask for a scratch.

The call button is wonderful in theory, but when it is out of reach, it's totally useless and only adds to the stress. At this time, I could do little more than turn my head, so if the call button was on my pillow and slipped beyond the radius of my head turn, I was helpless. Since the pillows were very smooth, this often happened.

... A First Step ...

The change in the nurse-to-patient ratio was rather dramatic for me. In Intensive Care, it was 1:1 or, at the worst, 1:2. In the Rockyview Medical Ward, I estimated the ratio to be about 1:4 or 5, but in practice it varied, depending on circumstances and time of day. This made sense, as the patients on that floor were not critically ill. In the rehabilitation ward, though, where patients were not routinely in need of any medical treatment, but only required teaching and assistance with daily living activities, it would be 1:4 on days, reducing to 1:5 in the evenings, and 1:8 at night. This meant that even if the need were urgent, there could be as much as a one-hour wait—which invariably seemed like two hours. Murphy's law would no doubt have it that if your call button were to slip out of reach when trying to alert the nursing station that your roommate had just fallen out of the window, it would happen straight after such a visit.

Sylvia's journal introduced nurse Norma, always smiling and cheerful, and physiotherapist Brenda, who was usually assisted by a very capable Marlon. To complete my therapy team, the occupational therapist was Nancy, ably supported by Elizabeth.

If the subsequent excerpts from Sylvia's journal contain only a few references to individual nurses or support staff, it is basically because I no longer had a nurse allocated exclusively to me. In this phase of my rehabilitation, however, I was fortunate to have some very caring and attentive nurses, most of whom had a good sense of humour, something extremely important for someone in my situation.

Now back to the journal:

Feb 17
S. Diary The wheelchair was altered and the leg supports improved to give Brian more comfort. In the interest of preventing bedsores, his mattress was changed to match the one he'd had at Rockyview.

Feb 18
S. Diary Daily stretching exercises started. Brian is left alone for long periods of time, depending on staff availability. He has his call button on his pillow, but

he gets stressed when it slips out of reach, which can happen in a matter of an inch or so.

Feb 19

S. Diary Brian got new hand splints, but no exercises were given, which bothered him. Hopefully they will start next week.

Feb 20

S. Diary Brian was bored today. There is no physiotherapy or occupational therapy over the weekend. I thought the nurses were quite sharp with him, and he responded similarly. He knows what he can and cannot do. No doubt this is an indication he is getting better.[32]

Feb 23

S. Diary Brian wants to discontinue the tablets he has been taking for diabetes. He thinks he is clear and is undergoing blood tests for a week, just to check. Another battle to get him back to bed ensued after lunch. He was in pain in his chair, and it took both of us complaining to get the issue resolved. They say they have had GBS patients before, but it sure does not seem like it. I was stressed and so was Brian. We don't need this.

* * *

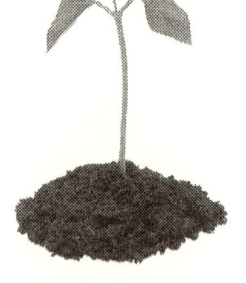

19
GBS Patients Are Neither Quadriplegics Nor Brain Damaged

In the rehabilitation ward, there seemed to be the previously encountered belief among a few of the staff that GBS patients could be treated as though they were quadriplegics or had spinal cord injuries.

Quadriplegics are those affected by paralysis of both arms and both legs. If the quadriplegia was incurred through a spinal cord injury, the trunk will also be affected. GBS, on the other hand, is usually characterized by general muscle weakness and paralysis. The essential difference is that, unlike the quadriplegic, when the GBS patient leaves Intensive Care and enters the rehabilitation ward, the recovery phase has commenced, allowing him or her to experience sensations that, although not altogether normal, do cause real discomfort.

I recall a number of assisted bowel routines when serious discomfort was experienced in the process. Rightly or wrongly, I believe the care provider did not realize I had regained almost full use of my stomach muscles.

It occurred to me, that those on the nursing team unaware of the distinction lacked an understanding of the discomfort suffered by the GBS patient, and were, consequently, sometimes reluctant to help reposition him. "You were turned only half an hour ago," was an oft-heard reply. Some seemed to have an unwritten rule that a patient could only be turned every two or three hours. Fortunately, they were in the minority. The overwhelming majority bent over backwards to ensure patient comfort.

Then there were those-again definitely a minority- whose actions demonstrated that they didn't realize that GBS patients were not brain damaged. This was partly understandable, perhaps, because a good number of the patients in the rehabilitation ward were brain damaged to a greater or lesser extent, either as a result of an accident or a condition such as a stroke.

I am hopeful that hospital staffs everywhere will understand that this is not criticism, but merely information not readily available elsewhere and will use it to glean a better understanding of the GBS patient's needs. This is particularly important in view of the patient's limited ability to communicate.

I cannot recall when the sensation in my trunk, arms, and legs actually returned. I do know, though, that by the time I was moved back to Foothills, if when lying on the bed, my legs were not in natural alignment, they soon hurt. When sitting in a wheelchair, I would often experience discomfort in my legs. This was no doubt due to nerves and muscles coming back.

During my stay in the rehabilitation ward, I was very much aware of shortages. There were shortages of nurses, of nurse's aides, and of equipment. The funding that hospitals in our province relied on had been subject to cutbacks, and this showed in so many ways, not the least of which was the time it took a nurse to respond to a patient's call. Undoubtedly, there were too few nurses, and those there were had to struggle to keep ahead. The stress showed, and that was unfortunate because there were some sterling people on staff who were trying very hard to do a good job.

There was another side to this, though. I was extremely fortunate to have been a resident of Alberta, in that the provincial health care plan covered the total cost of my hospitalization. For an individual living in another country without such medical coverage, I imagine the cost of seven months in Intensive Care would have been staggering.

Back to the journal, and good times enjoyed while working out:

Feb 24
S. Diary Brian had a much better day. He is working his arms in occupational therapy. Nancy, and her assistant Elizabeth were his therapists.

Feb 25
S. Diary Brian has experienced some chest pain. He had an x-ray to determine if he pulled a muscle or cracked a rib.

Feb 26
S. Diary More occupational therapy. Brian was in better spirits and is enjoying the challenge. He is using his shoulders more and working with arm slings.

Mar 1
S. Diary Brian is out of bed in chair for over six hours a day. He feels his needs are being addressed more.

Mar 2
S. Diary Brian has been named 'smiler' by some of the rehab patients. His diabetes tests were negative, and he no longer takes any medication except what is needed to keep him regular.

Mar 4
S. Diary A good day. Brian is doing well in both his occupational therapy and physiotherapy sessions. He was very cheerful.

Mar 5
S. Diary A home assessment was done, and we have some alterations to make before Brian comes home. Back at the hospital, he had another occupational therapy session, but the fact that oxygen was not put in his 02 cylinder wasn't noticed by the nurse

until after he got back to the room. No problem though-the hand-held Pulse Oximeter was reading 91-93.

Mar 6
S. Diary Brian was off oxygen from breakfast until around 4:00 when I left. Again, the Pulse Oximeter read 91-93, and there were no signs of stress-another step forward.

Mar 8
S. Diary Brian's tracheotomy was removed around 11 AM At his request, the doctor very kindly phoned to let me know it was going to be done. Later Brian was worried about coughing and wondered if the nurses would know how to handle him.

Mar 9
S. Diary Brian felt easier about his throat and was coughing less. He now has to hope that the opening left at the trachea site will heal on its own.

Although it is getting better with time, as muscles come back, coughing and sneezing have been difficult for him to accomplish successfully. Not all the muscles needed to perform a 'cough or sneeze' have been functioning, and this was particularly evident when he sneezed. The resulting sound was similar to that produced by a young child!

Mar 10
S. Diary A good day for Brian. He had a new chair and was very cheerful. The patient care manager just told him he may be allowed home for a couple of hours on Sunday the 14th.

Mar 12

S. Diary   Brian coughed a lot, but was clearing his throat successfully. The trachea site appears to be healing up a little.

Mar 13

S. Diary   Brian was quite drowsy early on, but perked up later. His oxygen reading was only 84, but improved to 92-93.

* * *

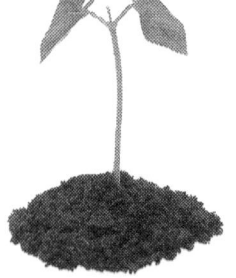

20
A First Visit Home

I was surprised, but very happy to be given a five-hour pass to go home. I never imagined this would happen so soon after being transferred to a rehab ward.

It had been a long time since I had seen my home, and there were a lot of emotions. It was incredibly good to be there with my wife and the family and our wonderfully helpful neighbours, most of whom were on hand to welcome me. On the negative side, I still had to carry oxygen, and that was somewhat intimidating. I was in a wheelchair, and experienced considerable discomfort, but knew I had to put up with it while my muscles and nerves were coming slowly back.

Most unusual sensations of discomfort, which are typical in the hands and feet, do disappear over time. I recall my hands being washed in Intensive Care and feeling like there were rocks in the sponge, but that sensation diminished over time. By the time I got to the rehab ward, there was much less discomfort, and a few months later that sensation had virtually disappeared.

Back to the Diary, and Sylvia's descriptions:

> **Mar 14**
> S. Diary A red-letter day! Brian came home for a visit! For the first time in over eight months, I have him home with me, even if only for five hours. I thank God we are winning at last. Sally accompanied him from and back to the hospital. It was a tiring day

... A First Step ...

for her and Kim too, but how we both appreciated it. Brian would have loved nothing better than to stay. He hopes to visit again next week.

Mar 15
S. Diary Brian is already planning to get home permanently and earlier than originally thought. He will need a special airbed and the right care.

In the hospital, he had his hair cut today; everyone noticed, of course!

Mar 16
S. Diary Another good day. Brian was excited to tell me he may be home both next Saturday and Sunday, but not overnight until we have the right kind of bed to prevent bedsores.

Mar 20
S. Diary Brian was home from 3:30 to 8:30 PM We had supper together at home for the first time in almost nine months. It was Brian's favourite, lamb and mint sauce. What a great feeling!

Mar 21
S. Diary The first day of spring, and it was beautiful. Again, Brian was home for about five hours. We phoned many of our relatives, and they were so pleased for us. Brian was relaxed and enjoyed the day.

Mar 23
S. Diary The new battery-powered electric wheelchair arrived on trial. If Brian chooses to keep it, he should enjoy much more mobility and independence.

Mar 24
S. Diary Visited early to join Brian in physiotherapy. I was

··· *A First Visit Home* ···

shown how to use a transfer board so I can get him from bed to chair when he is home.

Mar 27
S. *Diary* Better days ahead. Brian was home for about four hours.

Mar 28
S. *Diary* Another visit and, with assistance, I successfully transferred Brian to and from the bed.

Mar 29
S. *Diary* Muscle movement was detected under Brian's kneecap.

Mar 30
S. *Diary* Brian is trying out a new bed on the ward. Early signs are that he likes it.

In physio today, he was allowed to stand up for a couple of minutes with minimal support. His knees ached a little, but he was impressed with his accomplishment, as was everyone else.

* * *

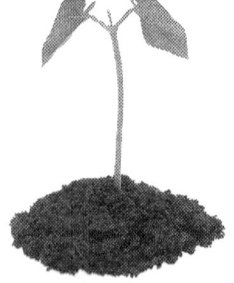

21
Some Reflections on Life in the Rehabilitation Ward

※ ※ ※

Easter is a time of hope and aliveness. For me, the early days of spring are, perhaps, the most exciting of the year with their promise of new life in the fields and gardens. To Canadians of the Prairie Provinces this was 'green-up' time and spelled more time out of doors, not to mention golf. From the window in the sitting area of my room, I could see one of Calgary's more established residential areas, school fields, and, at a distance, the Bow River with its paths and parkland.

From my bed at the opposite end of the room, where I had to spend quite a lot of time, all I could see were windows and concrete walls. I spent long hours pondering all the out of door activities I was missing.

Not that life inside the hospital was without its fun. I seem to recall an occupational therapy session towards the end of March when my therapist Nancy was experiencing a particularly busy week. I was in the OB sling (no one I have asked could explain what OB stands for!), which enabled me to move my arms free of gravity. I was also in a wheelchair. My exercises finished, Nancy duly started to put the sling away. Unfortunately I was still attached! We were to laugh about that many times.

Most of my physiotherapy and occupational therapy sessions were fun-filled. We were continually finding things to joke about. I was

A First Step

worked hard, no question about that, but with a great attitude, which, hopefully, I reflected.

A typical day started with a blanket bath followed by physiotherapy consisting of lower body stretching and range-of-motion exercises, which I did in my room. Then came breakfast. I had to be fed, since I was unable to move my hands-and although I did not know it at the time, it was to be two more years of conscientious exercising before I would regain significant hand movement.

No sooner had the remnants of breakfast been cleared away when my occupational therapy assistant Elizabeth would enter my room with her cold hands. I was convinced she warmed herself by working on me, and we used to laugh at that too.

After OT I could relax for about an hour; then I would be dressed and made ready for the morning physiotherapy session in the gym. The therapists, having already ascertained my personal goals and broken them down into smaller attainable ones, would put me through my paces. To make any kind of progress, it was necessary to practice the same activity over and over-things like standing upright on the tilt table and working on transfers, which entailed sliding on my buttocks on a smooth surface from a bed to a wheelchair and vice versa.

There were a multitude of obstacles, most of them small, and I had to work really hard at such things as getting back elbow range so I could touch my face. I recall the excitement generated on achieving such goals. No matter how minor, they represented huge steps on the road back. We saw every minute achievement as a huge victory.

When one has not yet regained the ability to walk or to stand up from a sitting position, using a transfer board requires superhuman effort, or so it seemed to me. It helped a little when I was transferring to a surface that was lower than where I started, since I'd get a little help from gravity. Unfortunately, there was always the other direction to master on the return trip. Either way, a therapist's assistance was still needed. Skill at transferring was important because eventually there wouldn't be two or three trained people around to help, and Sylvia would be assisting me, perhaps by herself.

··· *Some Reflections on Life in the Rehabilitation Ward* ···

After therapy, there was usually a less than an enjoyable hour or so before lunch would be served in the ward dining room. I always found that time somewhat boring. We were discouraged from getting back into bed, which was the most comfortable place to be, particularly after a good workout. This was to encourage wheelchair tolerance, but also because there wasn't enough time; so I would be left parked in the wheelchair, either in my room or in the small TV lounge. Occasionally, I'd have them bring me to the dining room so I could get a spot by a window. Since I was unable to use my arms, wherever they parked me, that's where I had to stay.

One of the worst parts of the rehabilitation phase was my almost total reliance on others. If I were to be wheeled somewhere and left, I would be totally reliant on someone noticing me or on my limited ability to attract attention before I could be rescued. In my room, it was a little different in that I always tried to ensure I had access to the call bell, and that made me feel less helpless. The need to get back in control was a large factor in my determination to beat GBS

Lunchtime was another adventure. Like many others in the rehabilitation ward, I had to be fed. I was lucky, since my wife would try to plan her visits to include lunch.

After the meal, I could relax for a while. Usually it was back to rest in bed until it was time for the afternoon therapy session. I tried to stay awake during this rest period, but usually succumbed to the sand man, proving myself a bad host to my very patient wife, who busied herself with knitting or reading-anything to make me feel less guilty, I used to think.

Invariably, I would just be falling into a deep sleep when I'd be woken up and made ready for my mid-afternoon occupational therapy. This would involve the usual exercises and required my practicing the same activity over and over. It was hard work, but I knew if I were to get my life back in my own hands, both literally and figuratively, hard work was what it was going to take.

On completion of the therapy session, I would be wheeled back to my room to await supper, at which time I was invariably fortunate enough to have the company of Sylvia, or sometimes my daughter Sally with my granddaughter Sarah, eagerly volunteering to feed me.

Now back to Sylvia's Journal, recording more progress:

Apr 4
S. Diary Easter Sunday. Brian was home for three hours yesterday and for supper today. Because he is spending more time in the wheelchair he is experiencing some discomfort in his legs. Today it is the left leg behind the knee and in the ankle area. He is eating better and enjoying home-cooked food.

Apr 5
S. Diary Everyone is impressed with Brian's progress.

Apr 7
S. Diary Both Nancy and Brenda saw movement in Brian's left wrist. This is wonderful news.

Apr 8
S. Diary What a great day! Brian had an EMG test, and his nerve responses in the left arm, wrist, and hand were positive. He was quite emotional — overwhelmed would be a better description. All the nurses were happy for him. The positive result means that, although he still cannot move his hands, he will soon be able to, as the nerves continue to repair. I was on cloud nine.[33]

Apr 10
S. Diary Home for six hours.

Apr 11
S. Diary Brian was home again to enjoy his favourite supper-lamb and mint sauce. He's talking about coming home for an overnight stay sometime soon. I wonder if we are ready for that?

Apr 13
S. Diary   Brian did a few arm exercises without the supporting frame. It tires him out, though.

Apr 16
S. Diary   Brian's arms are doing so well that, with help, he was able to scratch his eyebrow. He told me that he will be staying overnight next week, with home help arranged. A great feeling!

Apr 17
S. Diary   Today was our Wedding Anniversary, and Brian was home on a day pass to enjoy a family supper. I had a beautiful gift from him. Then our neighbour, Raymond, built a ramp so that Brian could move with ease in his wheelchair from the kitchen into the family room. It was so kind of him. It was a really enjoyable day.

Apr 18
S. Diary   Another day at home for the patient. He was with us for just over six hours and is looking much better.

Apr 20
S. Diary   Brian was excited to be driving a power wheelchair around the ward and then around the block. The doctor gave him the thumbs up as he went by.

Apr 21
S. Diary   Meeting with the Rehab doctor. He explained where we were at regarding Guillain-Barré and the rebuilding of nerves. He was still unsure of the recovery time, but I don't doubt that he was impressed with Brian's progress.

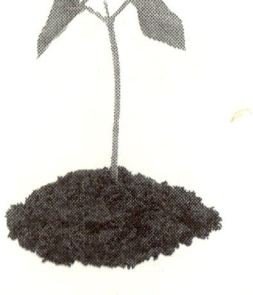

22
Was Guillain-Barré the Best Name for This Syndrome?

⁎ ⁎ ⁎

The more I thought about Guillain-Barré Syndrome and it's name, the more I believed, with apologies to Doctors Guillain and Barré, that a better name would have been 'Landry's Ascending Paralysis.' Importantly, it actually describes in straightforward terms what happens-typically, paralysis originating in the lower extremities and ascending up the body.

I understand the 'Miller-Fisher' variant of GBS does not necessarily follow this pattern; but since it, unlike other variants, affects the central nervous system, the Miller-Fisher variant could perhaps have been described as a different disease.

Further, with the descriptive name attributed to Doctor Landry, one would not have to keep spelling out G-U-I-L-L-A-I-N-B-A-R-R-E or continually tell people how to pronounce it. I feel sure it would have made life easier for doctors and nurses, as well as patients.

> The first clear description of the syndrome now attributed to Georges Guillain and Jean-Alexandre Barré was written back in 1859 and published in the French scientific literature, not by these two authors but by Jean Baptiste Octave Landry (1826-1865).[34]

··· A First Step ···

At the time the function of the peripheral nerves was not understood but Landry's beautifully descriptive account details all the key features of GBS. Landry was both a young man and a brave one. The patient (he was attending) was not under his care but under the management of his superior at the time, Dr Gubler. Landry records that Gubler mistakenly assumed that the patient was hysterical and, even in those days, recording the mistakes of your superiors cannot have been the way to advance your position! Gubler gallantly added a note to the report acknowledging that Landry had correctly predicted the demise of the patient at an early stage. Landry's patient developed difficulty breathing and in the absence of any form of respiratory support subsequently died. Landry found several other reports in the literature of similar cases and such patients became known as suffering from 'Landry's ascending paralysis'.[35]

After his description of 'ascending paralysis', Landry did not contribute any further reports to the medical literature (perhaps Gubler did take his revenge after all!) but set up in a successful practice involving hydrotherapy. He is said to have married a beautiful but poor wife (she obviously made him work too hard for the luxury of academic medical reports) eventually dying at the young age of 39 of cholera. He was reputed to have been extremely elegant and accomplished at dancing, singing and playing the cello.[36]

Maybe I would not be dancing, singing, and playing the cello during the coming weekend, but at least I would be home overnight for the first time. Sylvia goes on to describe the visit:

Apr 24

S. Diary Brian home for the weekend, including overnight Saturday. This was a first! He was in good spirits, but with the home-care aide, we really had no time alone.

Apr 29

S. Diary Attended a family conference at the hospital, which included Brian, the rehabilitation team, and the rehab doctor. It was basically a progress report and a spelling out of the changes needed at home before Brian could be discharged-tentatively set for May 20! One of the conditions is that he must have a hospital-type airbed so as to minimize the possibility of bedsores.

Apr 30

S. Diary Home again for the weekend-this time with overnight stays both Friday and Saturday. It was a noisy and busy time, both with visitors and attending to Brian's needs.

May 3

S. Diary We had a good day overall. I am getting great help from Sally, who is taking care of so many of the arrangements for Brian's homecoming.

May 4

S. Diary Brian came home again tonight to check out a trial bed. It was just an overnight visit.

May 8

S. Diary Home today and tomorrow for just a few hours due to the bed situation.

May 12

S. *Diary* Discharge date delayed to the 27th to allow time for the necessary alterations to be completed at home. In the mean time, there will be a lot of mess and dust-an unsuitable environment for Brian.

...

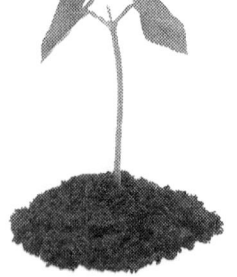

23

Changes Needed

We had to arrange for several changes to be made to our home in order to make it possible for me to live as normal a life as possible upon discharge from hospital. This, as so many things at this time, fell on Sylvia's shoulders; but, in spite of her inexperience in such matters, she coped very well.

Our home has two stories. At the ground level there is one step down to the family room, half bath, and garage entrance. Our neighbour had already kindly installed a ramp to give me access to this lower level by wheelchair. This meant that initially I would be limited to the ground floor; but even so, significant changes were needed to make that area liveable for me.

Most importantly, I needed access from outside. There were four steps leading to the front door, which made that entrance out of the question, or so we thought. That left the attached garage. Someone mentioned an elevator. After some thought, we decided it could work, enabling me to enter through the garage and ride up to the ground floor family room. The existing half bath wasn't suitable, so it had to be expanded into a full bath. We had just barely enough space to enlarge the area to include a shower.

Giving me access to the deck, lawn, and garden at the rear required widening the patio doorway. These alterations were the source of the 'mess and dust' that Sylvia referred to in her diary:

May 14
S. Diary An elevator was installed in the garage today to pro-

vide access for Brian's wheelchair. He is one step nearer to being independent. I was very tired after visiting today. There is so much to think about and do.

May 15

S. Diary Brian is home again for the weekend. We have a good caregiver for about two hours each day, so that helps me relax.

May 17

S. Diary These were difficult days for Brian. So close to his homecoming; it must be frustrating for him.

May 20

S. Diary The new hospital-type airbed was delivered. It was quite a day, to put it mildly. With all the phone calls and paperwork to look after, crazy may describe it better

May 21

S. Diary Brian was in really good shape. Did a couple of stand-ups for me at physio. He is still very shaky, but Brenda and Marlon left him alone-no hands-for a few seconds.[37]

May 22

S. Diary The building alterations needed to bring Brian home have been started. This involves re-doing the main floor bathroom and creating access to the deck and garden. It appears his discharge date is to be postponed again, as the way things are going, the alterations will not be complete by the 27th.

...

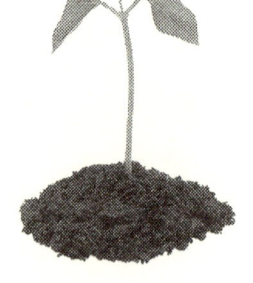

24
The First Steps

"I was never supposed to walk again, was I?"
"No you weren't, but then you don't listen, do you?"

I will long remember May 27. I went to the gym for physiotherapy, expecting nothing out of the ordinary. My daily session was at 11:00 AM and usually lasted an hour or, if I were lucky, a little longer. Brenda my physiotherapist must have had something on her mind. She suggested we go over to the parallel bars and said I should try to stand. As I wheeled over, Brenda positioned herself in front of me with a walker. Marlon and another assistant positioned themselves on either side of my chair.

With their help, I stood up and reached to the walker for support. After lying on a bed and sitting in a wheelchair for almost a year, standing erect gave me a feeling of exhilaration.

Now I know what Brenda is trying to have me do, I thought.

But I was wrong. That was not all. "Try to take a step forward," she said.

I tried. I tried so hard. My left foot moved slowly, then I put my weight on it and inched the right foot forward. I cannot describe the feeling of joy as I then put my weight on the right and shuffled my left foot forward another step. I seem to recall taking three steps in all that day.

I looked Brenda in the eye and said softly, "I was never supposed to walk again, was I?"

"No you weren't," she replied, "but then you don't listen, do you?"

"Brian, you've walked!" exclaimed Marlon. There were several onlookers, and I don't think there was a dry eye anywhere in the gym.

··· *A First Step* ···

Rumour has it that after my session, one physiotherapist ran into occupational therapy proclaiming, "Brian is walking! Brian is walking!"

Back to Sylvia's diary, where she describes that day from her perspective.

May 27
S. Diary   A wonderfully day! I saw a very excited Brian, who told me he had walked for the first time since getting GBS He took his first few steps on the parallel bars during physiotherapy. He also moved from the bed to his chair using a transfer board.

In occupational therapy, Nancy thought she noticed a flicker of movement in his left hand. That was two wonderful things taking place, neither of which may have been seen if Brian had already been at home. Wonders never cease. Thank God for helping us.

May 28
S. Diary   I spent time telephoning friends and relatives passing along the great news of Brian walking for the first time since Guillain-Barré Syndrome struck him down exactly eleven months ago today.

May 29
S. Diary   Brian is very content to be home again for the weekend. There is noticeably more strength in his arms and legs. He is happy with my planting of the garden, and the rainy weather has certainly helped the seeds. We are getting more organized with the caregivers.

May 31
S. Diary   Brian walked eleven paces in his physiotherapy session today! On the home front, alterations for his

homecoming are moving along, although, understandably, not fast enough for him.

Jun 3
S. Diary Brian's discharge date now appears to be set for next Monday, the 7th. I brought most of his things home from the hospital in anticipation of his release.

Jun 5
S. Diary Home for the weekend again. Brian lifted his right arm against gravity and touched his face for the first time.

Jun 6
S. Diary A good day for Brian. He was very content, although he could not get his legs comfortable. He may have been in his chair for too long yesterday.

* * *

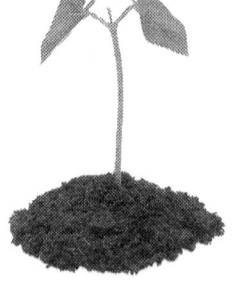

25
Homecoming

June 7th. This was the big day, the day I would get to go home. After over eleven months in the hospital, I was finally able to start living again. In addition to my wife Sylvia, my daughters Ruth, Kim, and Sally were there to greet me.

Sylvia recorded:

> It was a dull, cold, cloudy day, not much like June. We left the hospital at 1:45 PM, ironically with a Handi-bus driver who was having a bad day — or did he just have an odd sense of humour?[38]
>
> Brian was thrilled to be home. We had his favourite supper — lamb and mint sauce. Now there is so much to do, to arrange, and to remember. The alterations to the house are still ongoing. Home Care has so far been very helpful. I guess I was feeling overwhelmed. We have been through so much.

As for me, it was just great to savour the knowledge that at the end of the day, I did not have to go back to the hospital. It was an incredible feeling to know that, although I would, of course, be heavily reliant on others for some time, I would be in charge of my own life, at least in some respects. I still needed help with all those day-to-day things like feeding, getting dressed, being pushed around in the manual wheelchair loaned by the hospital. At least in important matters, though, I was now in control of my own destiny.

A First Step

My power wheelchair had not yet been delivered. It was custom designed to enable me to control it with my right shoulder-one of my few body parts that was working. Getting back to normal physically would take a lot of hard work, but I was lucky. I had a wonderful wife and family, as well as some devoted caregivers. Even as an outpatient, I was still able to rely on both my occupational therapist and physiotherapist, in whom I had full confidence.

Using Sylvia's Diary as my source, I will record further important developments in my recovery.

Jun 14
S. Diary Brian walked 35 paces in his physio session. Flickering can now be seen in his hands and wrists.

Jun 16
S. Diary Brian's wrists and fingers are noticeably moving. He had a heavy workout in physio, where he walked in the bars, not in too straight a line, but it is progress.

Jun 21
S. Diary Brian walked with the aid of a walker. It was difficult, but he felt good doing it.

Jun 25
S. Diary His hands are moving now-all fingers in unison. He can't yet move them individually. He held a ball.

Jun 30
S. Diary The tracheotomy site is still open, although the opening has closed to the size of a pinhead.

Jul 2
S. Diary Brian covered 100 metres on a walker in the gym.

Jul 7
S. Diary Brian folded his arms across his chest-another first. It might seem like a small achievement, but for him this was a huge step.

Jul 14
S. Diary Today, for the first time, Brian transferred himself from chair to bed unaided. That is really going to make life easier.

Jul 16
S. Diary Brian worked hard at physio and bade farewell to Brenda, who is taking a new position. She has seen so much improvement in Brian and helped so much.

Jul 19
S. Diary Today we took our first walk outside with Brian in his power wheelchair. He needed his safety belt on to remain centred when going over the many bumps.

Jul 22
S. Diary We took advantage of the good weather and went for another walk. It proved somewhat tiring for Brian's steering arm, but he will soon get used to it. He steers the wheelchair from his right shoulder.

Jul 26
S. Diary Good physio session. Brian is getting stronger, and walking and standing are now a little easier.

Aug 2
S. Diary Brian is moving his arms more, is able to turn the TV on and off, can turn the pages of the newspaper and scratch his nose, although the latter with

great effort. He is starting to get involved in business matters.

Aug 7
S. Diary   Today Brian was able to turn the pages of a book on his knee.

Aug 9
S. Diary   Julianne is Brian's new physiotherapist. She is very keen.

Aug 16
S. Diary   Brian weighed in at 135 lbs., up from 123 lbs. one month ago.

Aug 18
S. Diary   Brian's occupational therapist Nancy tried to help him put his hand to his mouth so he could feed himself. He didn't manage to do it during the day; but by evening he had succeeded.

Aug 23
S. Diary   Nancy added a one-pound weight, and, using his elbow, Brian raised his arm quite high. Julianne had him walk twice round the small gym, then stand by himself for a couple of minutes.

Sep 2
S. Diary   Brian transferred from the bed to a chair without my help and later transferred back again.

Sep 3
S. Diary   Most nights now, Brian is only waking up for turning and bathroom twice instead of three or four times.

Sep 11

S. Diary We were invited to a Lobster Fest at Brian's old company. It was great for him to see everyone again. The weather was cool, but at least we had sunshine.

Sep 15

S. Diary Brian handled the television remote much better.

Sep 22

S. Diary Julianne gave us some disappointing news: We may not see full recovery of the legs. Brian appeared not to be worried. He just said, "I don't accept that; I know she is wrong." His physio sessions are being reduced from three a week to two, which does not really please us.

Sep 23

S. Diary Brian's spirits are high and that keeps mine up, too. We will do exercises today and, God willing, will prove Julianne wrong. His feet-especially the right one-are beginning to cause him some discomfort. Perhaps that is a good sign.

Sep 28

S. Diary Holding a fork in a splint, Brian fed himself. He also used a calculator. He is so determined to prove everyone wrong. He is moving to and from the bed easier. If only his feet would wake up a little, it really would help.

Sep 29

S. Diary Brian weighed in at 130 lbs.

Oct 4

S. Diary Brian can now use the walker without help. He did

three laps around the gym with rest breaks. He is standing more securely and his knees are getting stronger.

Oct 5
S. Diary Brian can now hold his hand level without it drooping at the wrist when he raises his arm. His walking is improving.

Oct 7
S. Diary Brian feels it won't be too much longer before he can stand up from a sitting position without help. He is in really good spirits and feeling stronger every day.

Oct 13
S. Diary Nancy, Brian's occupational therapist, told us his elbows were greatly improved. She admitted to having believed he would never reach this far. This was reassuring for both of us.

Oct 22
S. Diary Brian moved the middle finger on his right hand and used it to start the power wheelchair himself. This was another first.

Nov 1
S. Diary Physiotherapy is going well. There is a definite improvement in Brian's ability to stand and sit back down. He lowers himself with much more control now.

Nov 5
S. Diary Again he weighed in at 130 lbs.

Nov 15

S. Diary Brian did his first 'walkabout'. With just a little assistance, he raised himself from sitting on the bed and got into the walker. His daytime caregiver Giselle and I stayed close by, just in case he needed help. He was pretty emotional. It was quite an achievement.[39]

* * *

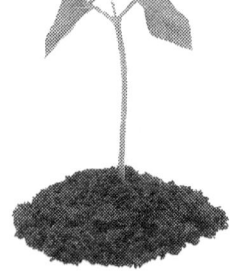

26

Starting to Live Again

It was now five months since I became an outpatient, and in spite of the large number of handicaps I still had to overcome, life was starting to get back to normal. There was little movement in my hands, and when not in the wheelchair, I still relied heavily on the walker to get around. This did not stop me. When I was not exercising or wrapped up in my physiotherapy, I was going forward with a new business venture; and I purchased my first computer to facilitate communication. Although I could not write, I was able to type with one finger.

I purchased voice-activated software, but soon gave up on that. Either the computer didn't like my English accent or my dictation was not clear enough for the software to handle. I spent more time correcting the errors that were continually occurring than on creating new work. I was fortunate, though, in knowing I would eventually have more use of my hands. This is what led me to dump the voice software. Otherwise, I would just have had to put more effort into making it work.

The new computer was not only great therapy, but it also gave others a break from having to constantly meet my emotional and intellectual needs. It kept me out of their hair. My daytime caregiver Giselle volunteered to teach me computer basics. This book is testament to her success. The last time I had used a computer was many years earlier in the punch card era, the steam age of computers, as it were. This was totally different.

A First Step

The picture for my wife and family also changed some. I still had to be fed and watered; and even with outside help, there was still a huge burden, particularly on my wife. I have the greatest admiration for her unfailing support and care and for her stamina. A lesser person would have been overwhelmed.

Just like anyone else, I occasionally succumbed to colds and the flu. Shortly before Christmas, I was sick and had to take a break from physiotherapy and home exercising. The timing was unfortunate since just as I was able to resume exercising, the physiotherapy, and occupational therapy units closed down for the Christmas break. I think this break in the therapy regime may well have delayed my recovery by more than a few weeks.

Shortly after New Years, the hospital cut my therapy from three times a week to two. I suspect this decision had been under consideration for some time and believe I have my therapists Nancy and Julianne to thank for keeping it unchanged until the New Year.[40] They had also encouraged me to make contact with a community physiotherapist and to follow up with fitness exercises at the University of Calgary.

Upon later reflection, I understand I was reaching a stage where improvements in my condition were such that some reduction in therapy could be made. Adding to or even maintaining the full therapy program would not have brought about any significant change; whereas the exercise program I was following at home would help increase muscle flexibility and strength. I realized the emphasis was starting to change from physiotherapy to exercising.

Christmas proved to be a much happier event than was the case last year. I was home, and it was great to have all our family visiting over the holidays. Then it was back to work-or rather exercising.

Before the first week of January was over, I had my first fall. I guess it was inevitable, but that did not make the experience any less uncomfortable. It happened in the bathroom, and I couldn't get up, so just had to lie there until help arrived. Fortunately, within a half hour or so, my niece Cara and her rugby-playing husband, Jamie arrived. Within seconds, Jamie had lifted me up and placed me on my feet, just like it was something he did every day.

··· *Starting to Live Again* ···

The next step in physiotherapy was literally a step upwards. I was helped to climb up two steps in the hospital gym. I had a hard time lifting my feet, but I had to start somewhere. Then a few days later Julianne introduced me to crutches.

I had to learn everything from scratch. My muscles had been out of action for so long that they had forgotten how to work. The fact I had been walking since the age of one made absolutely no difference. Walking, talking, swallowing without aspirating, and so many other taken-for-granted things had to be relearned. Things were starting to happen, though, and day by day, almost imperceptibly, changes were occurring. Little things, like being able to raise my left wrist or bend the knuckles on my left hand a little were encouraging signs of recovery. This was exciting, and I knew that improvement in a particular muscle on one hand or leg or ankle would be followed eventually by the same improvement on the other.

I also knew, in defiance of the prognosis given by many, that if my wrists and hands were coming back, then so would my ankles and feet. It was a little more than eighteen months since I was struck down, and though I still had a ways to go, I was continuing to see improvements.

Then the day came when I could raise my right wrist. A simple thing, but it felt so good.

It was now February, and Sylvia and I were advised that my outpatient occupational therapy would end in one month and my physiotherapy in two. This decision was reached even though there were still so many things I could not do. Now it was up to me to make the most of my last weeks as an outpatient.

Stair climbing was the top priority. Once when two physiotherapists were helping me climb stairs, I used the walker to get out of the wheelchair and then, with help, proceeded up the staircase sideways. To onlookers, it must have appeared that here was a crazy character who'd parked his wheelchair at the bottom of the staircase and was struggling to climb the stairs, needing the assistance of two therapists. To our amusement, a number of people passing by paused and, in all sincerity, pointed out that there were elevators just around the corner.

*** A First Step ***

To continue with my rehabilitation, with the emphasis now on strengthening, I was accepted into the University of Calgary Health and Fitness Program for the Handicapped. Most of my muscles-even the ones I was using-were fairly weak. The U of C program was precisely what I needed.

When I first saw the running track in the university gym, I knew immediately that I would not rest until I could run around it. I had no doubt that it would perhaps take years of hard work before I could accomplish that feat, but I was inspired.

Now, each step of my journey along the road to recovery brought more improvements. They weren't such big ones these days, but how do you keep matching momentous occasions like talking or walking for the first time? Even so, every little change was important. The first time I was able to move my little finger independently of the other fingers I wanted to tell the world.

Little by little, I recaptured my life: I walked on crutches outside of the parallel bars; I started being able to pick up some food with my hands without wearing a splint; with the help of physiotherapists, I practiced getting up from the floor after having fallen; and I walked outside for the first time with the aid of a walker.

By the end of March, twenty-one months after my initial brush with GBS I climbed stairs at home (with assistance) and entered my second floor bedroom. Then I went outside and was helped into the passenger seat of my car-all firsts! These achievements were important, particularly considering I was within one week of my last physiotherapy session as an outpatient at the Foothills Hospital.

Signing my own name, holding the telephone receiver, and picking up a sandwich were all firsts I celebrated in the following weeks. One of the most important improvements occurred in May. For at least a month, I had been able to use the muscle that pushes the foot down, but, in my opinion, that was not so useful or important as being able to use the opposing muscle, the tibialis anterior. One morning while doing my usual foot exercises, muscle movement was observed as, with assistance, I raised my left foot. I was particularly excited because this was a muscle I had been diligently working on ever since being discharged from hospital almost one year ago. Now, for the first time, it was flickering. This small movement was so critical in developing the ability to walk normally and drive a car. It was doubly exciting because the prognosis for it coming back had not been good. Now it seemed my months and months of effort had paid off- or perhaps it would have come back anyway. I will never know. The important thing was that it had.

I often wondered about how different my progress would have been had I believed those medical professionals who gave me little chance of recovery. In a disease such as GBS pessimism is most definitely the enemy. This cannot be emphasized enough.

In my case, because of my love of a challenge, it may have helped me. It certainly made me more determined to prove the doubters wrong. It did, however, make matters worse for my wife and family, especially in those early days when I could not communicate. I had not been aware just how bad my prognosis was; but even if I had been, I was unable to tell them to ignore the bad news and believe in my ability to recover. In my own mind, I never doubted for one second that I would get well again. They, on the other hand, had to live with the fear until I disproved it.

I have since learned that mine was the most severe case of GBS most of those medical professionals had seen. They could not have known what a fighter they had on their hands. More than one family member tried to convince them of that fact, but we easily become the victims of our preconceived notions.

I continued to slowly make progress in a number of different areas. As the weeks passed, I was starting to move all my fingers independently and could make a complete 'O' with the finger and thumb of my right hand. I stood at the kitchen sink to have my hair washed and used an electric razor. So the shaving wasn't perfect; but it was a start.

Then I found I was able to grip some heavier objects and lift them. One morning two and a half years after losing the use of all my muscles, I was lying on my back in bed and moved my feet up and down. I was stretching my whole body. It suddenly dawned on me that I was actually moving my ankles totally unassisted. I was thrilled.

I kept setting new goals. These would include graduating from

A First Step

a walker to a cane, getting free of the wheelchair, and climbing stairs without assistance. I knew these skills would not come overnight and that I would have to work very hard; but the goals would be worth achieving. Then it would be on to gardening and, ultimately, to golf.

I will get back. Stay tuned...

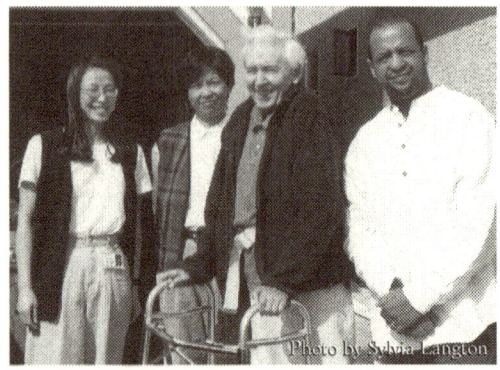

Left to right; Julianne, physiotherapist; Cindy, caregiver; the Author, and Marlon, assistant physiotherapist. The physiotherapists had visited my home to help me get into my car for the first time since hospitalization.

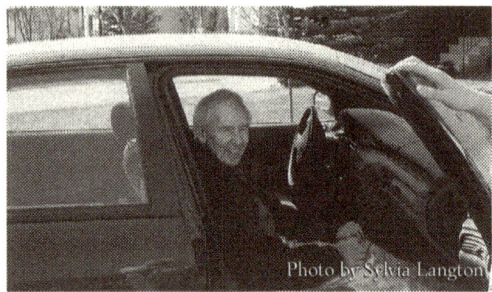

Mission accomplished!

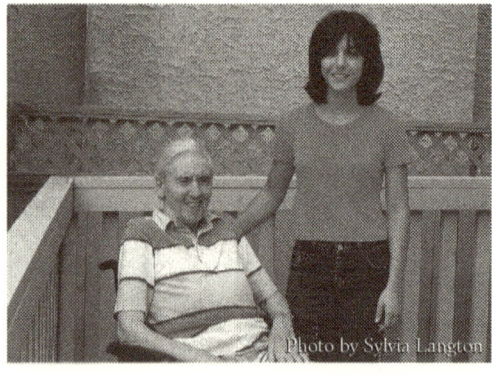

Giselle, caregiver, right, and the Author.

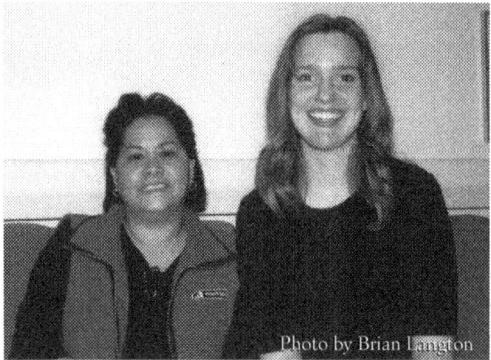

Nancy, occupational therapist, right, and her assistant Elizabeth.

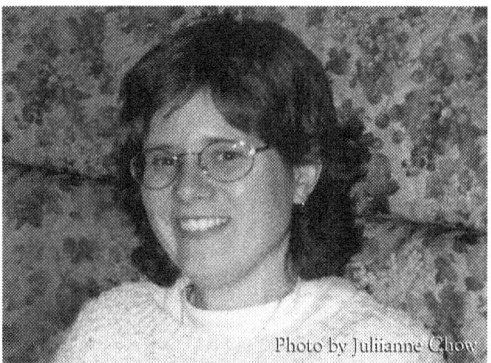

Physiotherapist, Brenda, enjoying a well-earned break.

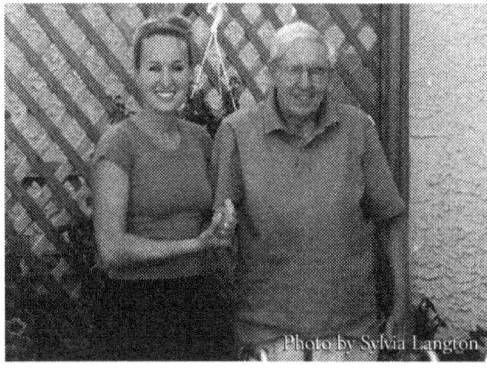

Another first! The Author making the break from his walker, with caregiver Tara offering her arm in support.

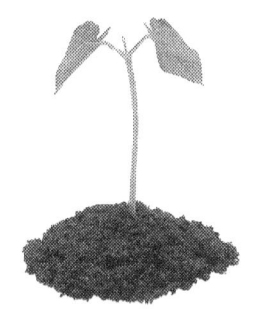

Part II
In Dreams...

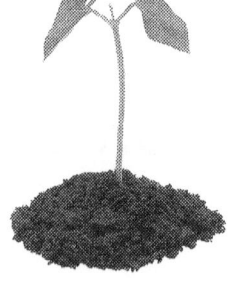

Intro
Dream Sequences

• • •

During my extended confinement in Intensive Care, I experienced many dreams and hallucinations, some of which are described here.

You may wonder about their place in this book. I chose to include them for three reasons. Firstly, because the stories seem to me to demonstrate how the brain managed to remain active in a body it no longer controlled. Secondly because of the important role the dreams played in helping me, the patient, keep a sense of humour, and provide a more light-hearted environment for both myself and those visiting. Thirdly, there are important messages within the stories for interested medical professionals and care providers, enabling them to identify the underlying needs of a patient, in some cases contradicting previously held beliefs. One example, as a patient, I craved attention in any way I could get it. I did not ever want to be left on my own. Whatever it took to gain the attention of the nursing staff, whether by means of flashing lights, alarms, or other noise, was all preferable to the 'calm, quiet and orderliness,' for long thought to be desirable in an Intensive Care ward. This, I believe, becomes clear as one reads the dream sequence 'Submariner in Trouble.' Then there is the sequence, 'Jet Fighters on Call.' The reference to the outside view providing the basis for this story, underlines the need for 'a room with a view,' to challenge the mind of a long term intensive care patient, and allow for contact, even if only visual, with the outside world.

In relating the stories to family and friends visiting during the later part of my stay in hospital, I quite often had the listener in hysterics. This then gave me a feeling of well-being, which, in the circumstances was invaluable, and proved such a morale booster to everyone concerned about my situation, given there were still many hurdles to overcome.

A First Step

No effort has been made to determine the trigger for the dreams. I don't even know if it is possible for such a determination to be made. The medications I was taking, albeit rarely, the inability to distinguish between night and day, being thrust into an unfamiliar environment, or something inherent in the disease itself may have been the cause. Although these dreams are not necessarily in the sequence in which I dreamed them, it is possible to connect some of them to certain events or phases of my illness.

I found these episodes much more intense than the garden-variety dream. In fact, most seemed so real that sometimes it was difficult, if not impossible, to separate them from reality. Every effort has been made to keep to the original story lines. It must, of course, be understood there were a few — although very few — grey areas, and only in those situations have I linked different parts of the story by the logical threads suggested by circumstances. For the most part, my recall of these dreams was total.

Except for my relatives, the names used to identify characters are fictitious and used to enable the reader to follow the thread of the story. In these sequences, any similarity to any person, living or deceased, other than in the case of the exception noted, is entirely coincidental and unintended.

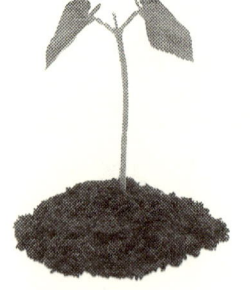

27
GBS Patient on a Secret Mission

I was enjoying the spacious surroundings at our weekend cottage in Calgary. It was on a lot in a very quiet subdivision, and its back garden bordered the land occupied by the Hotel Deluxe. The funny thing was, I could only vaguely remember how to get there.

The hotel itself was a fine piece of architecture ten stories high, with the usual swimming pool between the rear of the hotel and my property. It was good to have a pleasant area next door.

As I was relaxing in the cottage garden on this particular day, I could see a group of three people-two very smartly dressed businessmen and a very attractive young blonde woman, whom I assumed to be a sales person-at one of the hotel's umbrella-covered tables. They were looking and pointing in my direction, as though I were the subject of their conversation. I thought I recognized one of the men as the director of a government department interested in publicizing and obtaining support for Guillain- Barré Syndrome patients and their families.

It became very clear that I was the topic of their conversation when the three of them got up and started walking towards the gateway that separated the hotel from my cottage. I beckoned them to come through to join me.

I now knew I had correctly identified one of the men as Manny Olafson, the director. He had once provided tickets for Sylvia and me to go on two short vacations as part of the healing process. He had then turned around and used me for his own publicity purposes, which made me feel very foolish because I was displayed in a tight-fitting neck brace. I did not want to be used in such a distasteful way again.

The three came over to where I was sitting, and the person I recognized as Manny introduced me to his colleagues Tommy Tomlinson and Grizelda Fredericks. As I expected, Manny offered me another trip, but this time it did not include Sylvia. He refused to name the destination, but suggested I would enjoy the time away from the hospital. Remembering the last two trips and believing the purpose was again a publicity stunt, I refused.

Manny, however, would not take no for an answer. He used every argument he could think of to try to persuade me to accept his offer. Finally, he could see he was getting nowhere and got up to leave. Tommy and Grizelda left with him.

Now, I thought to myself, *I can relax and enjoy the sun with the knowledge that I do not have to put up with anymore of Manny's distasteful publicity trips.* Little did I know that they were not about to let the matter drop. This became clear when Grizelda appeared again at my gate. I had no alternative but to invite her to join me. She continued pressing me to accept the trip that Manny was offering, arguing that in view of everything that he and his colleagues were trying to do for me and fellow Guillain-Barré sufferers, I should have the decency to at least consider his offer. She reminded me that they were solely interested in raising funds to improve awareness, treatments, and research.

Again I said no, and Grizelda could see that I was adamant. Indeed I was. If Sylvia wasn't included, there was no way I would accept. At this point, Grizelda's demeanour changed. "What if I can persuade Manny and the department to include Sylvia? Would that make a difference?" she asked.

I thought for a few moments and, with a feeling that I might live to regret my decision, agreed to go. I told her it would also be nice to know where we would be going. I was a little concerned about the secrecy and wondered why it was necessary.

She left to talk to Manny and, maybe an hour later, returned with confirmation that the department had agreed to allow both Sylvia and me to go on the trip. She could not, however, let me know the destination.

The next morning, just as I was about to enjoy my coffee in the garden, who should appear but Manny looking very pleased with himself. "I'm glad you have agreed to go on the trip, but please, mention this to no one. You will understand why later," he said. Still puzzled by the secrecy, I reluctantly agreed. By this time I was starting to suspect I was dealing with the government. Again, I asked about the destination, but all Manny would say was that I shouldn't worry and I would be advised later.

I spent the next few days relaxing, although the forthcoming trip was on my mind and I was making sure we would be ready to leave on short notice.

Then one morning Tommy Tomlinson arrived with one of his colleagues, a man named Peter Woodward, whom I'd not met before. "Okay, let's go," said Tommy. "Everything has been arranged. We have your tickets here, and Sylvia's will be delivered to her separately since she will be meeting up with you later."

With that, we were off to Southport Road in Calgary. For readers not familiar with Calgary, Southport Road is a narrow street bordered by trees and an arterial roadway on one side and buildings of perhaps eight stories on the other. When we got there, a shining new Boeing 737 was waiting. Tommy and Peter helped me board the plane, which was full. This surprised me since it was supposed to be a top-secret mission. Tommy assessed the situation and told Peter to go to the tail section and try to make room for an extra seat. I'm not sure how he accomplished this, but somehow he managed. With me rather awkwardly seated between Tommy and Peter who were standing, Tommy signalled that we were ready for take-off.

I had experienced some white-knuckled take-offs, but none like this one. With the engines roaring and Tommy and Peter holding me in my seat, the plane was in the air. Or was it? We seemed to climb a bit, but then dove and levelled out with the office buildings at eye level. Then we climbed again, and the captain came over the intercom and apologized, saying the rough take-off was caused, no doubt, by the extra seat in the back!

⋯ A First Step ⋯

"Okay, where are we headed and where is Sylvia?" I asked Tommy.

"Don't worry. Sylvia will be meeting up with us later. I am only cleared to tell you that we will be landing at Red Deer International Airport," he answered. (For those not familiar with Red Deer, Alberta, there is no international airport anywhere close.) "All the passengers are obviously aware that we are flying into Red Deer," Tommy went on, "so there was no secret about this part of the journey. I will let you know our ultimate destination when we take off on the next leg."

The landing at Red Deer was a little bumpy, but otherwise uneventful. After the other passengers had disembarked, I was led into the airport building. Peter said we should go to one of the offices in the customs area and he would then explain the purpose of the trip and provide me with some important information. Tommy added that Manny would meet us there. One of the customs officers recognized Tommy and pointed to one of the offices, indicating that we would not be disturbed.

When we got to the room, Manny was there, along with another familiar-looking person who had the sort of face that you see on television many times but cannot put a name to. Manny welcomed me, said he hoped I'd had a good flight to Red Deer, and introduced the other man as Minister of the Department of Foreign Affairs and International Trade. The minister shook my hand warmly and said he hoped I would be up to the mission they had in mind for me.

"Mission?" I asked, "You said *mission*, not *trip*."

The minister looked a little embarrassed and said that the nature of the journey had not been disclosed for security reasons. He apologized and gestured us to sit down at a large table.

"Even now," said the minister, "I am unable to tell you the exact destination; but you are headed for a developing country and will be part of a very secret mission-so secret, in fact, that before leaving you will be required to sign a waiver signifying that you will not admit to having any connection with this country and that you will defend the government against any claim for any reason whatsoever. "Also," he went on, "I have to tell you that, should you be captured and taken prisoner, the government will deny any knowledge of you.

The purpose of the mission is twofold-to support freedom fighters fighting for democracy and to create greater awareness of the Guillain-Barré Syndrome, which does not distinguish between people. As we all know, GBS is a very rare condition. You are one of the few people currently afflicted, and you were chosen because you are capable of supporting a better understanding of Guillain-Barré. This is a politically sensitive area, and the utmost security must be observed. We are aware of at least one foreign power that, to put it mildly, would take great exception to our presence in that part of the world. What do you think, Brian?"

Dare I tell him that I felt very taken advantage of, but also thought it might be fun? It was a little like being on a roller coaster-once the thing starts, there's no getting off until the ride is over. "Look," I said, "I don't appreciate being kept in the dark, but I do understand the reasons for it. Yes, I will accept a place on the mission, providing Sylvia can join me. But I must know when she and I can meet up."

"Good," said the minister. "I will make a phone call after which I, hopefully, will have an answer for you."

Sylvia, meanwhile, was shopping with our daughter Sally. Just before they were about to return home, Sally remembered she had to make a phone call. She parked and went in search of a pay phone, leaving Sylvia alone. As soon as Sally was out of sight, two secret service agents approached, showed their identification, and asked Sylvia to accompany them. They explained that they would be taking her to join me, but for security reasons, her disappearance had to look like a kidnapping.

Sylvia protested, but her efforts were to no avail. The agents reminded her that national security and the safety of the mission were involved. With that, they quickly ushered her to a waiting sport utility vehicle and drove away.

"I have spoken to Ottawa," the minister said, turning to face me, "and understand that arrangements have been made for your wife to meet you at the top-secret overseas staging area in Okotoks, Alberta. We shall be flying there in about two hours. We did not go there directly because flights from Calgary would surely be tracked on radar by the foreign powers interested in the developing country we have targeted. Flights out of Red Deer will not be monitored or attract attention. For our mission to succeed, we have to ensure the utmost secrecy. In the meantime," he continued, "I must ask you to sign this waiver, which apart from freeing the government from all liability for anything which might happen to you, requires that you not carry modern medicines or anything else that would indicate that you are not a citizen of our target country."

I was particularly alarmed at the notion of being without antibiotics because I had pneumonia. The thought of having to wait until my return to North America to resume my treatment, or worse, of becoming sicker while overseas really scared me. I discussed my concern with the minister, but could see I would get nowhere. "All right," I said finally. "Pass me the documents and I will sign. I am committed to the mission and will see this through, but I'd really like to know who will be traveling with me and what relevance this mission has to publicizing the Guillain-Barré Syndrome?"

"Sure," replied the minister. "In addition to the crew, you will be accompanied by approximately forty others, including engineers, technicians, mercenaries, and a medical staff of five. There will be two doctors on the team, and it will be their responsibility to arrange for visits to hospitals and clinics when we arrive at our destination-which you will be advised of when we reach the overseas staging area in Okotoks. You and Manny will leave in about an hour. Sylvia and the others will be arriving there independently. I hope this answers your questions."

"Fine," I said. "That is good to know."

In less than an hour, Manny and I were on an old DC3 for the forty-five minute flight to Okotoks.

Our landing was uneventful, considering the age of the plane. As we disembarked, I thanked the pilot; then we proceeded to a building in the staging area. Security was very tight. I said goodbye to Manny and was ushered by an agent of some kind through a maze of corridors to an office in a large hangar-type building, where I was asked to wait. After about ten minutes, a nurse came in and told me I was going to be given a medical examination and checked out for any modern drugs or antibiotics that may have been in my system. She said that I shouldn't worry; I would be made comfortable.

At this point, two men came into the office. "Hello, I guess you are Brian," said one. "My name is Alan, and I would like to introduce you to Lieutenant Colonel Randolph Hillier, the commanding officer of the staging unit."

"Hi Brian, I am pleased to meet you," said the lieutenant colonel, "Please call me Randy. I know are wondering where we will be sending you. Your destination is Boravia, and you will be accompanied by a number of dedicated professionals, including the medical people with whom you will be working-if everything goes well, that is. Do you have any questions?"

"Yes I do have questions. I presume the mercenaries with whom I am traveling will be responsible for our security en route, but what happens once we land in Boravia? Will we be on our own?"

"Pretty much," Randy admitted. "That's why when you get there, it will be important to blend into the local community as well as you can, avoiding, where possible, any connection to our country. We cannot appear to be sending in an independent security force. You will be visiting several hospitals and clinics with the medical team, but, as for the mercenaries, they have other business."

I told Randy I understood, at which point he said he would leave me for now so I could proceed with my medical exam.

As he and Alan left the office, the nurse reappeared and called for an assistant to bring in a stretcher. Some stretcher! It was more like a trestle table on wheels. At least it had a thin mattress to make the surface a little more bearable. I was helped-or more accurately, lifted-onto the table and left while the nurse went to prepare the equipment necessary for my exam.

As I would have expected, it was at least half an hour before she returned. In the meantime, Alan came in and told me he had an invitation for me from the chief. "There will be an F-16 fighter jet on the airfield tomorrow morning, and he wonders if you would like to fly it."

"You bet I would," I replied.

"Flown before?" Alan asked.

A First Step

"Only as a fare-paying passenger. But I would be happy to give it a try."

Alan then explained that the F-16 would be available at 10:15 AM and that the wing commander would give me a run through of the flight controls. He added that he would come for me about 7:30, allowing enough time for him to help me into my flying gear.

All this time the nurse had been standing by, not sure whether to laugh or cry!

Now I was in her hands. As she started on my medical, I mentioned that I felt my pneumonia was getting worse and questioned her about my prospects if I were unable to continue taking antibiotics. Her response was that old-fashioned remedies had been available before antibiotics and that appropriate ones would be issued to me. Surprisingly, this satisfied me.

At about ten the next morning, complete with my helmet, oxygen kit, ejector harness (which I had struggled with), and the rest of my flight gear, I made my way onto the airstrip and noticed an older Boeing 757 sitting at the edge of the runway. Its paint was worn away, and it looked somewhat worse for the wear. *I hope we're not flying to Boravia in that*, I thought. Then I saw the F-16. It was either fresh from the factory or newly painted. The wing commander had just arrived, and when he saw me, he came over to give me a cheery welcome to his wing, which consisted of three F-16's.

"Okay, let's get on-board," he said, "and I'll show you the controls. It all looks terribly complicated, but I enjoy flying these birds and think you will, too. Just think. If you bring your F-16 back safely, you will probably go on record as the oldest pilot to fly one!" I smiled at this and then began paying very serious attention to everything he was showing me in the cockpit.

The 'flying lesson' completed, the wing commander suggested I make myself comfortable behind the controls, keep my hands clear of the canopy as it closed, go through the pre-flight checks, and prepare for takeoff. The tower gave me permission to head to the main runway as soon as I was ready.

Taxiing to the designated runway was not too difficult, and the experience gave me quite a bit of confidence, most of it probably false. I just had to make sure the F-16 did not get away from me and soon learned to apply just enough of the brake to keep her in check. *Boy, this is not so bad*, I thought.

I soon mastered changing directions and turning. Learning as I went, I reached the runway and radioed the tower for permission to take off, which I was promptly given. There was no other traffic in the area. Now came the big test.

I allowed the 'big bird' to start rolling forward. Gradually at first, then suddenly, tremendous 'g' forces were pressing me into the back of my seat. This was exhilarating. I increased power and was soon hurtling down the runway. Then, after gently easing back on the stick, I was airborne.

After successfully flying around the area for about half an hour, I decided to bring the aircraft back to its base and hoped I hadn't forgotten all I needed to know to land her safely. It was now white-knuckle time, as the runway appeared a lot closer than it should have been. Was it my speed or just the fact that I was not thinking quickly enough? I decided to go around one more time. I gently lifted the nose and adding more power. Again the F-16 responded much faster than I expected. I was starting to sweat.

This is it- the best approach I can make, I tried to convince myself. It was like being at the top of a hill on a bicycle without any brakes. Gently I eased the craft around, feeling it was controlling me rather than the other way around. I persevered, however, and lined up with the runway, then cut back on the power and eased the plane down- if it's possible to ease down something that's travelling in excess of two hundred kilometres per hour. Closer and closer the runway appeared to be rushing towards me. I braced myself, fought to keep the F-16 from drifting to the left, and straightened up just in time to make a heavy two-point landing. Okay, so it was not a perfect touchdown. At least I made terra firma in one piece and succeeded in stopping just short of the end of the runway. Any spectators-and I'm thinking here of the wing commander in particular-must have been scared out of their wits!

On firm ground again, it was now time to return to the maintenance hangar and continue with my medical exam. I found myself

··· *A First Step* ···

back on to one of those uncomfortable stretchers and was quickly wheeled into another room, where I noticed a number of other people on similar stretchers, also seemingly preparing for their medicals. Then suddenly on the other side of the room, leaning up from her stretcher was Sylvia! She was waving madly to attract my attention. I had really mixed feelings. Don't get me wrong, it was great to see her there, but what had I got her into? No wonder "the department" and their spokesman Manny had resisted including her. At least I have to give them credit for keeping their word. "See you soon!" I called to her.

At this point, the nurse took control and put me through some gruelling tests. As she took a blood pressure reading, she mentioned having seen me land. "Enough," I said. "Let's not talk about that. It wasn't the best part of the flight!" She smiled without saying anything and continued with her work. While this was happening I could see that Sylvia was also getting medical work done.

The next morning the medical team, Sylvia, and I were given a briefing on the conditions we were likely to encounter at our destination, which we now knew to be Boravia. Since we had to avoid immigration and customs, we would not be landing at the capital. In all probability, the landing was going to be a rough one, but our agents in the field had assured us that the runway would be just long enough for our 757. While this was going on, we could hear jet engines being powered up.

We were going to have to live pretty primitively, but at least the temperature would be in the thirties (Centigrade). Captain Rob Jefferson, the briefing officer, asserted, "The nearest town or village is deep in the bush, some forty kilometres from our runway. A driver, who will have a Bedford truck at his disposal, will meet us; and from there, we will be making for Newport, the capital. To avoid any suspicion as to our identities, we are going to have to make it look as though we are simply entering the capital from within the country." With that, he wrapped up the meeting and asked us to be ready to board in two hours. "I will be with you as part of the medical team, so if there are any more questions we can address them on the flight."

After a farewell dinner in the mess hall, those of us who were departing for Boravia assembled in front of the main hangar and started to make our way towards a parked Boeing 757, freshly painted in Boravian Air colours. The forty or fifty people ready to board would certainly not fill the aircraft, but as we later discovered, a large number of seats had been removed for cargo and supplies.

Once onboard, Sylvia and I chose our seats-not in my favourite window position-and started to make ourselves comfortable. I could not help noticing that the condition inside the aircraft did not match the fresh paint on the outside, and the few seats were cramped and well worn. The interior design was from another age. It reminded me of the sixties! All around people were smoking, and I remember hoping that a "Please extinguish all cigarettes" sign would appear before takeoff.

The moment of truth had arrived. The jet's engines were revving up loudly now, and on came the signs-not only "Fasten seat belts," but also "Please extinguish all cigarettes." So far, so good. We started to taxi towards the runway.

Speaking as though we were all fare-paying passengers, the captain came on the intercom, welcomed us, and thanked us for choosing to fly Boravian Air. As he was drawing attention to the 'Fasten seat belts sign', his demeanour changed, and he suddenly exclaimed, "What idiot left an F-16 on the end of the runway?" I wished I were an ostrich and could have stuck my head in the sand to avoid my embarrassment.

The pilot must have had clearance, since the engines appeared to be almost at full power, and then we started to roll. All conversations ceased as we accelerated down the runway. A gentle bump, then a harder one, and we were airborne. I guess in the interim, some kind person must have moved the F-16!

We seemed to be climbing for a long time. The quiet that settled in during take off remained for some time. There was a good deal of turbulence, and it was really bumpy until we appeared to be at cruising altitude. Then normal conversations and joking around resumed.

Our flight, which from that point was uneventful, seemed to go on forever. I did not time it, but after what seemed like seven or eight hours, the captain announced that we were about to descend and that all normal formalities, including the fastening of seatbelts, should be observed. "The crew hopes you enjoyed your flight with Boravian Air and that you will fly with us again," crooned the captain's voice over the intercom. Except for a little more turbulence, our landing was fairly routine until we actually touched down. At that point the ride became quite rough. When we finally came to a standstill, we started to relax and congratulate each other on still being in one piece.

Rob Jefferson came over to where Sylvia and I were seated and explained that we would be exiting the aircraft with the medical team, including him, and leaving the others behind for their top-secret briefing. I do not have a clear recollection of how we disembarked. There was only a clearing in the bush, a single runway with no airport or other facilities in view. Who knows? Maybe we grabbed onto a tree and shimmied down to the ground. I rather suspect, though, that some form of ladder must have been deployed from the aircraft.

The group of us, consisting of Rob, two medical doctors, two medics, Sylvia and me, were by now standing just off the runway looking for any sign of the Bedford truck that should have been sent out to meet us. There was no vehicle to be seen. We decided that, for security reasons, the driver must have gone to some pains to keep the vehicle out of sight. If he did not come out of the bushes to meet us soon, we would have to go search for him.

To the west of the airstrip there was nothing but low scrub for some distance. No place for a truck there. The east side was a different story. It was a jungle with only two apparent clearings. The one immediately opposite us was the obvious first choice to head into to look for our driver.

It wasn't long before we spotted what we were looking for. There was the Bedford. Although it appeared some effort had been made to hide it at the side of the clearing, it didn't take us long to find it. But where was the driver? There was something odd here.

Rob and I went for a closer look. What we saw horrified us. When we opened the passenger-side door, there was a figure slumped over the steering wheel, his head covered in blood. One of the medics had joined us by now, and he felt for a pulse. There was none.

After further checks, the medic turned to us and indicated something we did not wish to hear-the driver had been dead for some time.

Now what? Here we were, miles from Newport confronting this grizzly death. Rob asked one of the doctors if he would drive. His name was Jock, and he was as Scottish as the misty highlands of that great country. "Of course," he replied without any hesitation. "Just give me the directions, laddy. I'll get you to Newport."

That being decided, we started to come to grips with the reality of our situation. We had to get our luggage off the plane, but first we had to give the unfortunate driver some sort of a burial. That took time, but we finally accomplished the sad task. Then it was back to the runway and the 757. We were in luck. The crew, and maybe others on the aircraft, had unloaded our equipment and supplies. Everything we needed was neatly stacked on the side of the runway. There was no activity, so we assumed the briefing was still ongoing on the plane. Jock drove up in the Bedford, and we started to load.

As soon as everything had been placed on board, we all climbed into the truck. Sylvia sat in the cab with Jock, while the rest of us made ourselves as comfortable as we could in the back amongst our boxes of equipment. Jock, looking very confident behind the wheel, turned to see if everyone was safely accommodated. A vocal chorus of "O-Kay lets go" from the five of us in the back was enough for him.

"Hold it," Rob called out to Jock. He was having second thoughts about Sylvia being up front and pointed out that her presence there could attract attention we did not need. Sylvia quickly agreed to abandon the comparative luxury of the cab and joined us in the back of the truck. Then we were off.

We drove slowly through the cleared area, which got increasingly narrow as we proceeded away from the airstrip. It was a rough ride and dusty too. This must have been their dry season.

Soon we came to another road, which could certainly not be called a main road, although it obviously carried more traffic than the one we were on. After a brief pause at the junction, we headed north towards Newport. The sun was getting lower in the sky and throwing shadows across our path. Suddenly, upon rounding a bend, we saw a roadblock. Two trucks were parked together, making passage through impossible. Standing around the barricade formed by these trucks were, perhaps, a dozen men. They appeared to be soldiers, and all brandished automatic weapons. Jock glanced quickly at Rob as if looking for directions on how to react, although he later admitted there was no option but to stop and hope we would be allowed through.

As we slowed and came to a halt just short of the barricade, the soldiers cautiously approached with their guns at the ready. The leader appeared to be a junior officer, and it was he who approached Jock and asked for I.D. One of the soldiers leapt on to the back of the Bedford, while the others encircled us. We anxiously awaited some indication as to whether we would be allowed to proceed. To our dismay, the soldier pointed his gun at each of us in turn and made it clear that he wanted our watches and any other valuables we may have had with us.

We had no alternative but to comply. Meanwhile, Jock was doing his best to convince the young officer that we had been transferring patients from Newport to the St. Augustine Auxiliary Hospital. He later said he'd recalled hearing that place name at one of his briefing sessions. The officer had obviously noticed the blood on the dashboard and lower section of the windshield, and Jock hoped his story would sound convincing.

"What sort of patients?" questioned the officer?

"Bleeders," Jock replied, and the soldier seemed satisfied. In the meantime, things were not going so well in the back. We were being relieved of anything the soldiers considered of value. Not quietly though. Everyone was complaining loudly, and that made our adversaries very nervous. By then, another two had climbed in and were helping to collect the loot.

Due to the noise we were making, no one noticed a northbound vehicle rounding the bend in the road behind us. Its headlights were off and it approached quietly and deliberately, pulling up a short distance behind us.

Suddenly, all hell broke loose. Our adversaries, so greedily involved in their hunt for instant wealth, found themselves surrounded by a large number of well-armed mercenaries, some of whom just happened to be our flight companions. The soldiers who had stopped us fired a few shots in panic and surprise at having the tables turned on them, then quickly saw they were outgunned and outnumbered. They handed our belongings back and grimly climbed down from the truck, where, following the lead of their commanding officer, they surrendered to the mercenaries. All of their weapons were confiscated and placed on the truck behind us. Round one to us.

A half dozen of the mercenaries left to take the now frightened soldiers into the bush. We were to learn later no lasting harm came to them. They were merely taken a good distance from the road, tied up, and left to their own devices. Meanwhile, Jock and Rob got to work moving the soldier's trucks so we could pass. Both vehicles were driven off the road into the bush. We were assured that the trucks were so well hidden, even if their attackers freed themselves and reached the road, they would have trouble finding them.

We all stood around for a while, talking and expressing our thanks to the mercenaries for their timely intervention. After saying their farewells, the rag tag group took leave of us, and with wry grins, suggested we keep out of further trouble.

I suggested to Rob that we leave this area and look for somewhere to bunk down some distance away. He agreed and asked Jock to load up and continue on our heading towards Newport while he kept his eyes open for some place to drive off into the bush and set up camp for the night.

The next day dawned extremely hot and humid. We gathered our belongings and clambered aboard our trusty Bedford. Jock checked to make sure everyone and everything was secure, and we were on our way. No one said anything, but we all realized that the closer we got to Newport, the greater the danger. We got within twenty kilometres of the capital. Then the rains came.

We hastily pulled the tarp over the back of the truck to cover our belongings and ourselves and concentrated on keeping dry as we sped along. Soon we left the densely wooded bush behind. Every now and again there were clearings with shanty-type buildings, some standing on their own, some in groups.

··· *A First Step* ···

By this time, I was feeling really sick. The hot, humid weather was making my chest condition worse. If only I could get some help at the military hospital in Newport. I was in dire need of a deep suction to drain my lungs of fluid. *How can I beat this pneumonia without antibiotics?* I wondered. Normally I hated the thought of antibiotics, but for something as serious as this they were necessary.

Even though we were now on the outskirts of the capital, the road was not in very good repair. We were really getting thrown around.

"There's the hospital," Jock called out, after rounding an almost-blind corner. It was an old, but substantial, building in a well-treed river valley. "We should make it in about five minutes," he added, driving a little faster now down the fairly steep hillside. Sylvia and the others had been discussing my condition and had decided they'd better change their original plans and get me into the military hospital as soon as possible. I was in no shape to argue.

"Okay, here's what we do," said Rob. "I've already talked it over with Jock. He'll drive us to a grocery store just this side of the hospital and drop off everyone except Brian. Then he will drive to the emergency entrance. This should not cause anyone to connect them with a vehicle containing seven people being sought by the military, if indeed the word about us is out. He will stay with Brian until he is admitted. Once he's situated, we can then visit. Is everyone happy with that? I don't think we have any other choice."

Was this the way I was supposed to be visiting clinics and hospitals in Boravia to publicize Guillain-Barré Syndrome? I wondered. As we were just about to drop him, and the other passengers, including Sylvia, at the supermarket, I put the question to Rob.

"No, not exactly", he replied, very apologetically. "Like everyone else, I'd hoped your pneumonia would have cleared up by now. Your Guillain-Barré Syndrome is more than enough for you to handle, but you know what governments are like with all the bureaucracy. They want us to push ahead, regardless."

With that, he jumped out and, Jock headed for the hospital.

The next thing I knew, I was surrounded by faces. I didn't recognize where I was, but knew it must be the military hospital. People were prodding me, lifting my arms and legs, enquiring if I could feel what they were doing, and asking a host of other questions. I hoped this would not go on for too long and that I would be able to get some treatment, if not for my Guillain-Barré, certainly for my pneumonia.

It's ironic, I found myself thinking, *Here I am in the hospital belonging to the same military who tried to rob us. We are trying to help their country, and what are they doing?*

Many hours with me fitfully dropping in and out of sleep. Then I heard a familiar voice. It was Rob. "Just relax," he said. "I am going to put you to sleep. We are going to help you and make you more comfortable." I started to thank him and ask to see Sylvia, but never finished the sentence. He had gently covered my face with a cloth soaked in ether. Sylvia explained what happened sometime later.

I could hear the unmistakable sound of jet engines. I thought I was on an aircraft, but I was in a hospital bed-or was it a stretcher? Since there was an intravenous feeding bottle hanging above my head. I decided it had to be a stretcher. One of the medics came by. "What is happening?" I asked him. "Where are we going?"

"We're on our way home," he replied.

"But," I started to protest, "we haven't finished the mission yet, have we?"

"Yes sir, we have. You've been out of it for six days. It's all finished, at least as far as the medical side is concerned. Now, we're just hoping we have enough fuel to make it home. The captain says it's touch and go. We've already jettisoned the surplus equipment, including some aircraft parts, to lighten the load."

We were now on a 'white knuckle' flight for a reason very different from the norm. It's not often a shortage of fuel is the culprit.

The next few hours were tense for everyone, and surely for no one more than the captain and his co-pilot. Very little was said. The hours passed. Rob came by to check on me. "Where are we now in relation to Canada?" I asked.

"We just passed over Churchill, Manitoba," he said thoughtfully. Normally from Churchill, it's about two and a half hours to Calgary. I hope we can make it." I nodded my agreement.

Another hour passed, and the huge jet engines were purring

smoothly. It seemed impossible that anything could go wrong now. Then the dreaded announcement came, and behind the captain's voice we could hear alarms sounding in the cockpit. We all knew what was coming.

"This is your captain speaking," he said. There is even less fuel than our earlier calculations suggested so we're going to make an emergency landing. We have permission to land at a small airstrip which, given our present distance and altitude, we should be able to reach. It will likely be a rough landing, but we will do our best to get us out of this in one piece. Everyone please be seated and fasten your seat belts. When I announce that we're on final approach, please adopt the crash-landing posture, head between your knees." So this was it.

Rob came over to me with some webbing and proceeded to tie my stretcher to the plane's framework; then he fastened me securely to the stretcher. He was working quickly, but very efficiently. The last of the engines was shutting down, and then there was nothing but wind noise. It was quiet-eerie in fact.

Having taken care of me, Rob went to his own seat, sat down, and fastened his safety belt. We could all feel the descending motion of the aircraft. Sometimes it seemed to dive more steeply than at others. Everyone understood only too well that there was no room for error.

Minutes seemed like hours as we glided down from our cruising altitude. We waited. Then suddenly the co-pilot came into the main cabin just long enough to tell us to assume the crash position. "We have no intercom, and we are on final approach." After a brief pause, he added, "Hold on. We will make it. We have to." With that he went to rejoin the crew. I could only imagine what was going on in the cockpit.

One of the medics looked out the window. "Gee, we're coming in fast," he yelled. There was not much I could do. I figured I'd be lucky to survive this on a stretcher. I remember wondering if anyone had ever survived the rush of blood from the head to the feet that happens between 150 and 200 kilometres an hour.

There were a few minutes of quiet, a loud bang, and then nothing. I must have passed out. I had obviously survived the landing, but my head was swimming and I ached all over. I tried to get up to make sure everyone else had survived and to survey the damage. With great relief I saw Sylvia. She was all right and making herself useful bandaging Jock's leg. He had a nasty looking gash just below the knee. The cabin was a mess, but fortunately everyone seemed to be accounted for. The crew must have done a great job in getting the aircraft down. No fire had resulted, and we were able to organize ourselves and use the damaged cabin as a temporary headquarters.

Rob announced he was going to survey the airstrip and find out what facilities and equipment were available. Jock offered to join him, but had to back down when he put his full weight on his leg. Meanwhile, we raided the galley. It had been some time since our last meal.

"Good news and bad news," Rob called out as he clambered back into the cabin. "Which do you want first?" Without waiting for an answer, he continued, "The good news is there is an aircraft available for us to continue our flight; the bad news is that it's, an old biplane, an Avro Tutor. There are normally no aircraft on this field. We just got lucky. The Tutor had landed for refuelling. It's only a two-seater and has a full payload already-the pilot and his passenger- so we will have to hang onto whatever we can-struts, wing supports, anything. The pilot says if you can find a handhold, he will go for take off. He promises to fly as low as he safely can. The responsibility, though, is all ours. What do you think?"

"How long would we be in the air?" I asked. The Tutor can't have a very high cruising speed. I would hazard a guess it's somewhere between 100 to 120 miles an hour."

"You're probably right," said Jock. "And if that's the case, it's likely to take us about five hours to reach Calgary. Quite a long time to be exposed to the elements."

"At least the air is warm," Rob added.

Regardless of the obvious risks, and without much hesitation, everyone agreed to go for it. By this time, we all wanted to get home. I had been torn out of the webbing by the impact of landing, so now had to be lifted back onto my stretcher and then carried out of the cabin and across the field to where the Avro Tutor was parked. It looked in reasonable shape, to my novice eye, anyway.

The engine was still, although the pilot was standing by. He was, no doubt, conserving fuel for the last leg of our flight, which must have been close to the limit of the aircraft's range. We didn't need any more crash landings. I hoped he had calculated the additional weight he was to carry!

I was gently transferred from my stretcher onto the lower wing. My condition made it impossible for me to grip anything, so Jock bound me, as best he could, to the struts. Once I had been secured, Sylvia and the others found places where they could hold on. Sylvia lay on the lower port wing on the other side of the struts from me; and I saw one of the medics clamber onto the wing between Sylvia and the fuselage. The only grip he had was the leading edge of the wing, but I guess he knew what he was doing. Rob was trying to make himself comfortable on the tail section. I only hoped this bird would fly with all the 'interruptions' the presence of bodies on the flying surfaces would create.

"All right, we'll start the engine," the pilot announced as he clambered into his seat. His initial passenger, who we later learned was also acting as his navigator, was already in place. The Pilot had obviously arranged for take-off assistance, for just at this moment a late-sixties-model car pulled up alongside us, and two overall-clad men alighted. One had his eye on the chocks, while the other went straight to the propeller, and going through the usual hand start motions, commenced to swing. After four or five strong downward pulls, the engine burst into life, spluttering and backfiring a little at first, but finally settling into a steady rhythmic sound. The pilot made a quick final check of his controls and called for the chocks to be pulled.

Slowly he eased the heavily burdened biplane over the grass field toward the single runway. The old Tutor felt like it would fall apart at the next bounce. Luckily, it survived, and to everyone's relief, arrived at the opposite end of the runway from where our big jet had crash-landed.

There was no control tower here to give clearance, so everything was up to the pilot. He was obviously thinking hard about the jet he had to clear at the runway's end. Could he climb high enough in time?

After getting lined up, he taxied to a halt, then opened the throttle, and we were rolling, slowly at first, then at a speed one might expect to go on a Sunday afternoon drive. Our damaged jet was starting to look awfully close, but we continued down the runway. I could feel that we'd picked up a little bit of speed. The pilot had the throttle wide open, but we still weren't going fast enough to lift. Then, just as we passed the point of no return, it seemed we might actually gain sufficient height to clear the jet.

The pilot, with a lot of courage, waited until we were almost out of room, then pulled back on the stick and, almost without waiting to leave the hardtop, banked sharply to the left. We missed the jet by inches. We'd hardly gotten through that situation when up in front of us loomed an eight-foot fence. We were so low that it looked like we might not make it, particularly in our attitude, which the pilot quickly corrected and only just in time. Again, we missed disaster by inches.

We were gaining altitude now, but slowly. We had to hope there were no high-tension cables in our path for the next twelve miles or so. If there were, this journey could be over. The navigator should know, but if he did, he wasn't saying-not that those of us clinging to the wings would have been able to hear him if he had.

The air rushing by me was now a gale force wind. In addition to being bound to the struts, I was instinctively trying to curl my fingers around them to get a grip, but of course, it was useless. I couldn't move my hands. Even willpower could not overcome the paralysis. I did manage to give Sylvia a reassuring nudge, however. In return, she gave me a kind of a half smile, which told me she not only understood, but accepted the situation we were in. "I only hope we don't run into rain," I shouted to her.

Fortunately the weather was clear. There wasn't a cloud to be seen.

Suddenly there was a piercing scream. The medic holding on to the bottom wing near Sylvia must have lost his grip. There was nothing to stop him from sliding into the void. Our height couldn't have been more than fifteen hundred feet, but for the medic, it might as well have been fifteen thousand. We looked around and encouraged one another to hang tight. I saw Rob gripping the tail section for dear life and marvelled at the pilot's skill and the ruggedness of the biplane. I thought of Jock on the starboard side and hoped he had a good handhold.

Whether it was the warm air rising or the fact that we were one body lighter, we started to gain a little altitude. Good thing, as there were some fairly high hills in our path. At least once, the pilot had to take evasive action to avoid flying into one. It was fortunate for us all that those hills were not mountains.

I started thinking that maybe the medic whom we'd lost might be all right, after all. If he had fallen to earth as we were flying over a hilltop, he may have only dropped three or four feet, rolled over a few times and survived with nothing more than a few cuts and bruises.

For those of us still hanging on, cramps were beginning to set in. Everyone's hair was flowing straight out behind them in the wind current. Tiredness was becoming a factor. It was amazing more of us hadn't plummeted to the ground.

Hours passed. Areas of my upper body, which had previously started to show some movement, were now getting numb. Suddenly, the aircraft lifted noticeably, and I wondered if we'd lost someone else. I turned and checked for Sylvia. She was very tired, but so far all right, thank goodness. I looked behind, and Rob was still perched, albeit precariously, on the tail. It occurred to me that maybe someone on the other wing had gone to sleep and just slipped off into nothingness.

Now the Tutor was really starting to climb, and we no longer had to be concerned about high-tension cables or towers. We were flying over bald prairie, so hills were no longer in the reckoning, either. That was a distinct advantage; except we now had no hilltop to drop onto if we got tired and couldn't hang on.

In the distance, the Rocky Mountains were now visible. They were a wonderful sight because they signified we were finally reaching home territory. *Perhaps now*, I thought, *my pneumonia can be completely cleared up and the rest of my treatment or therapy continued. Hopefully the prognosis will be better.*

GBS Patient on a Secret Mission

Suddenly there it was, Calgary International Airport. Strong Chinook winds must have been blowing because we were coming in at quite an angle, but slowly. Our air speed may have been ninety knots or so, but we were only making headway against land objects at perhaps forty to fifty miles per hour. I was thinking about our fuel supply.

Suddenly, a body came falling down from the top wing, whizzing by just in front of my head and disappearing into the void below. We must have had more passengers than we realized. No wonder the old biplane had experienced so much difficulty getting and staying airborne.

The Tutor rose up-in response to losing some weight, no doubt-and then her nose dipped into an even more steep descent, which brought us down to maybe fifty feet above the runway. Boosting the power, the pilot held us in level flight for a few moments and then gently eased the aircraft down onto the runway.

We had made it-and without losing anyone else!

* * *

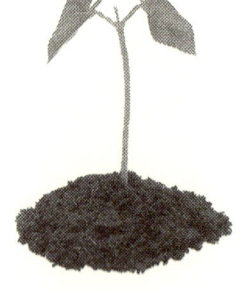

28
Who Wants to Buy a Double-Decker Bus?

※ ※ ※

It can be hot in Calgary in July, and this day was. Not yet eight in the morning, and it was already twenty-three degrees Centigrade. I'd just dropped Sylvia off to meet her friends and was driving with the windows down, enjoying the warm fresh air. I was in a part of the city that I wasn't familiar with, and when I noticed a turn leading to the foot of a gorge, I thought I would explore. After about a kilometre or so, the road started to rise quite steeply.

Now I was climbing to the top of the gorge. Suddenly, after rounding a tight bend, I saw a large notice at the side of the road: "Win $50,000 by having your car driven over the gorge at the lowest possible speed!" was the message. "Lose, and we take your car in exchange for a trade-in."

This sounded tempting. According to the notice, the lowest speed achieved so far was ten kilometres per hour. The camber of the road on the bridge was such that if a car actually stopped, it would surely fall off. For some reason, though, I was convinced that I could drive over it at seven kilometres per hour without taking a tumble. It would be close, but I could do it.

I pulled over when I saw a small wooden cabin with same 'Win $50,000...' poster. A young man was standing at the door. *Probably a summer student*, I thought. Upon getting closer, I decided he looked familiar. Then I was sure. "Your mother is a nurse at the hospital, isn't she?" I asked. He nodded. Now I knew I would get a fair deal here.

"All right, I'll buy a ticket and drive over," I asserted. "How much?"

"Just ten dollars" was his reply.

I paid him and looked to the gate, expecting it to be opened for me. Instead, the young man held out his hand and asked for my keys. My stomach tightened. "Why?" I asked.

"I have to drive you over. Those are the rules." Now I saw I had neglected to read the small print. *What do I do now?* I thought. I decided it was still a good deal. I didn't think the nurse's son would take unfair advantage, at least I hoped he wouldn't. When he agreed that I could ride with him, I gave him the keys and told him I was sure that it was possible to drive this car over the bridge at seven kilometres per hour. He nodded. Then, knowing I was beyond the point of no return, I moved over to the passenger side and relaxed.

Off we went. As we approached the bridge, we slowed down to about fifteen kilometres per hour and, to my dismay, continued across at that speed. "What do you think you're doing?" I yelled. "You aren't even trying! You can go much slower than this."

"Sorry" was all he would say!

Now I was getting quite angry. I knew I'd been taken for a ride in more ways than one, and I was beginning to feel very foolish. *How could I get taken in like this?* I asked myself.

We quickly reached the other side, where there was another small cabin attended by four men. One appeared to be a regular employee, but the others could easily have qualified as nightclub bouncers. Had I decided to dispute the result of this "slowest over the bridge" competition, there was no doubt in my mind as to who would win the argument.

"Your keys please."

My heart sank. The man I thought to be an employee handed me a document to sign. He explained it was required by the government to confirm both the sale of my car and the fact that I was trading it in 'voluntarily'! It was becoming very clear that there would be no getting out of this. The other three men-the muscle-bound ones-had moved to block my only means of escape. The alternative was a three-hundred foot drop.

I signed his waiver and looked at the receipt he handed me. I'd estimated the value of my car to be about $17,000. The receipt showed a value of $14,000, for which I would receive two trade-ins. One was a four-year-old import, dusty green, ill-kept and rusted, worth $6,000. The other, which I'd be told about later, was valued at $8,000.

I didn't believe how stupid I'd been! How could I tell Sylvia and my daughters that I'd gambled away our virtually new car? How could I admit to behaving so recklessly? And it wasn't only my family. What about the bank? I still owed money on that car. Not much admittedly, but the fact remained that there was a lien on it.

The next morning I awoke in the Intensive Care Unit, still connected to a ventilator and an intravenous drip feed. Nurses came and went, as did breakfast time and bath time. Or was it the other way around? I wasn't sure and could not have cared less. My problem was how to tell the bank manager!

Two days went by. Then one of the respiratory therapists came into my room and gave me a cheque for $4,000 dollars and a promissory note for, of all things, a Double-Decker bus. I was considering what it might mean as he gave me one of my regular suctions. *What was his part in this*, I wondered? And what could I do with a Double-Decker? I still had not phoned the bank, and this was worrying me more than anything else.

I spent all the next day trying to figure out how to phone the bank manager and what the consequences of that conversation might be. Since I couldn't use my hands, someone would have to dial and hold the phone for me, and that could only happen if a telephone were brought into my room in Intensive Care. That created another problem. Whoever held the phone could not avoid overhearing how foolish I had been. What a dilemma!

The following day brought more problems. After what would have been breakfast time for most people, but not me since I was on intravenous feeding, I happened to look out of my window. It was a beautiful sunny day with typical Alberta blue skies. Then I saw

··· A First Step ···

something that changed my day. A red Double-Decker bus-my Double-Decker bus-was parked on the road outside the hospital. I did not need this. Looking around, I could see the nurses were all occupied, so out of bed I leapt and hurried out of the hospital, hoping I wouldn't be missed. I ran right into the arms of the respiratory therapist who had brought me the money.

"I was hoping to see you," he said. "Here are the keys for your bus!"

Hardly pausing, I took them and continued out of the building. I had never driven a bus before, so things in the next little while could prove to be tricky.

Seeing the bus at close quarters brought all the earlier concerns rushing back to mind. I couldn't keep it, that much was clear; but how could it be disposed of? In the meantime it couldn't be left where it was because it was in a no parking zone. Then I had an idea. I had a friend who ran a small business in a subdivision of Calgary, and I thought perhaps he might have space for me to park the bus until I could decide what to do with it. *It's worth a try!* I thought.

I struggled into the drivers seat, made myself comfortable, and with some trepidation, turned the key. The engine roared to life. *Now to get this behemoth to my friend's in one piece!*

After a white-knuckled drive that took about thirty minutes, I arrived at my intended destination and swung the bus off the road onto my friend's unpaved forecourt, hitting a few potholes, which bounced the tall vehicle rather precariously from side to side, before coming to a halt. With relief, I wiped the perspiration off my forehead.

The feeling was short lived. Looking around, I failed to see any sign of activity. It appeared my friend had gone out of business or moved. Now what to do? I dared not leave the bus. What would happen if a construction crew was slated to start work here in the morning? I felt I had no option but to search around for a suitable road on which to park and just hope I could find someone in the next day or so who wanted to buy my bus.

I released the parking brake and carefully drove back to the road. After a few blocks, I noticed a rather wide road running off to the right. *Maybe this will do* I thought and signalled to make the turn. The road went uphill for a short distance, and although a number of cars were parked along it, there appeared to be a lot of space on the crest. Choosing my spot, I parallel parked the bus, set the brake, switched off the engine, and pocketed the keys.

After looking around to see if I were being observed-who would want a Double Decker parked in front of their house?-I made a quick exit, crossed over to the other sidewalk, and walked away.

It was time for my blanket bath. I had just woken up. Who had helped me back to Intensive Care and how? The hospital was a long way from where I left the bus. For a short time, my attention was held by what was happening in my room. Aides were changing the beds and one offered me a hot blanket, which I gladly accepted. No one seemed to have missed me yesterday. As soon as I was alone, my thoughts returned to selling the bus. I still had not phoned the bank!

The best way to handle a problem like this, I told myself, *is to do something about it.* The next time one of my daughters came in, I would ask her to pick up an 'Auto-Trader' publication and would use it to identify possible markets for the Double-Decker. This thought put my mind at ease. I could phone the bank later.

Several days later, my eldest daughter brought me the publication, which I gratefully put on my bedside table. This part was real. Several months later when we were reminiscing, she told me she had assumed I was looking at mini-vans capable of carrying a wheelchair.

After the visit, I asked the next nurse to come into my room if she would just flip through the magazine for me since I could not use my hands. After transferring me into the wheelchair with the help of five other nurses, she went through the book with me. To my dismay, there was absolutely nothing about any kind of bus, never mind a Double-Decker. Now I was starting to worry again. Time was passing, and I could imagine the parking tickets piling up.

I had to talk to the respiratory therapist who gave me the cheque and promissory note. "I need a suction," I told the nurse, hoping the right therapist would respond. I was disappointed. I had to wait two more days. When he finally came, I plucked up the courage to ask,

··· *A First Step* ···

"Could you help me sell the Double Decker that was traded to me? I have no contacts, but I assume you must have"

The respiratory therapist gave me a very strange look and, after a moment or two, took a step backwards and said, "Let's talk about that tomorrow." I was puzzled by his reaction. He seemed to want to wash his hands of the matter. The next few days of worrying about accumulating parking tickets, how to contact the bank, and whom to tell, passed very slowly. Visitors came and went, and to some extent they took my mind off my concerns. My wife was a constant companion, and I appreciated being distracted from the vehicle problems.

A day or two later, my daughter Sally happened to make a very significant comment. She and her husband were keeping their M.G. in our garage. The subject came up, and I asked her if it were now easier to move in the garage than it used to be. She looked a little quizzical, but assured me there was no problem with space. I pressed further and asked what she thought about the dirty, rusted old car I now had.

"Dad, your car isn't rusty," she said. "Admittedly it's quite dusty, but then it hasn't been used for some time. You can still see the colour of it, though. The green finish still looks good."

All of a sudden things came clear. Sally was, if I dared believe her, describing my car. If my car was still at home, then I couldn't have lost it in a stupid wager. More than that, if there had been no wager, then there couldn't have been any trades either! If there were no trades, then there was no bus and no horrendous quantity of parking tickets. I had been worrying for nothing.

My car was an Eagle Vision. Just to be really sure, I threw caution to the winds and asked Sally one more question. "What car are you referring to?"

"Your Eagle Vision, Dad. Why?"

...

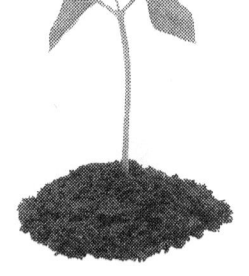

29
Submariner in Trouble

It was stuffy and dark. It was also late at night, and from the noises we must have been submerged, or so I thought. I was being accommodated in the hold of what appeared to be a large submarine. I didn't know how I got there or why, and it was impossible to ask, since I was totally unable to communicate. I was paralysed and totally reliant on the nurse in charge perceiving my needs. To expect answers to complicated questions such as "What am I doing here?" was not realistic.

I lay in my bunk, frustrated at my inability to move. A great deal of the time, I was uncomfortable. From time to time, instrument lights would flash, and occasionally, alarms would go off. Not that I minded the lights or the general confusion. Indeed, the more that was happening, the better my chances of being seen by a passing nurse.

My nurse, or at least the one I thought was mine, had a bunk in the same room. It had a drape, which could be pulled across for privacy.[41] Whenever someone's alarm sounded, she would pull back her drape, get out of her bunk, and go check things out.

On this particular night, I had a brick, or something that felt like one, in my bed. I was lying on it! Now, if only an alarm would sound, maybe the nurse would come.

Paralysed or not, I could use my eyes, or so I thought, to signal my extreme discomfort. Still my chances of attracting attention were not good. I don't know how long I'd been there, but I couldn't remember the last time anyone had spoken to me, let alone come to adjust my bedding.

Suddenly another alarm sounded. It wasn't mine, but it was close enough that to investigate it, the nurse would have to walk right by my bunk. Finally, I might get lucky!

At first, there was movement in her bunk. Then, her drape moved to the side, and in the half-light, I saw her get out of bed, hurry along past my bunk without so much as a glance at me, and fumble around with one of the other patient's ventilators. Now if I were to attract her attention, it would have to be on her way back.

I was really getting desperate. If only I could cause something to fall to the floor that she would have to stop and pick up or that she would trip over. Of course, since I couldn't move, that was out of the question. I had to think quickly. What else could I do? Maybe I could move my head from side to side to let her know that there was a problem. Unfortunately, just because I felt that I could move my head didn't mean I actually was able to. I was aware that what I thought I was doing wasn't necessarily what was happening.[42] Even so, I had to give it a try.

Sure enough, having solved the other patient's problem, the nurse returned to her bunk without even looking in my direction.

This would happen time and time again. I couldn't understand how the nurse could be unaware of my condition and my ongoing need of attention. Was she just choosing to do nothing? I can't remember how long I was ignored in this fashion or how I finally got out of the submarine.[43] I did, however, have the thought that I was no good to the navy while incapacitated!

...

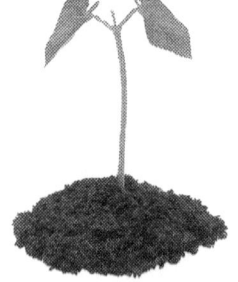

30
Guardian Angel in a Stetson

⋯

I awoke one morning to find an interesting looking envelope on my bed. I opened it and discovered an invitation to an open house being held the following week. Although I didn't recognize the sender or the address, I thought that I would have ample time to discover the origin of the invitation.

Sometime later, when a respiratory therapist named Don came into the room to suction me, I suddenly recalled that he'd talked about a friend who had the same name as the one on my invitation. I asked Don if he had been invited to a party, thinking this might tell me whom the invitation was from and, possibly, why I was included. He said he had been and added that the party was being given by a rather eccentric friend of his named Mike, who had a habit of throwing somewhat less than wild parties at his home in the country.

"I don't think I will be going, though," Don said. Then, "Don't tell me you have also had the misfortune to receive an invitation from Mike?" Obviously feeling guilty over his indiscretion, he added, "Don't take me too seriously; he's not a bad chap, really."

"Yes," I told him. "I've been invited, and I'd like to have a night out, so I think I will accept. Sure you won't change your mind and join me?" Don shook his head.

The day of the open house arrived. Since I had decided it was best not to go too early, it must have been about 8:00 or even a little later when I reached Mike's house. I cannot recall how I left the hospital, but presume I had traveled in or with my wheelchair. To my sur-

A First Step

prise, I was the first one there. Mike ushered me into to a fairly large lounge and asked me to sit down. The way the furniture had been arranged indicated that we were in for an evening of playing cards.

Before long, several other people arrived and briefly introduced themselves. One of them, Kenny, appeared to be quite the organizer and obviously knew his way around. All the other guests seemed to know each other.

By now I had sensed that this was going to be one long, boring evening. I have never enjoyed playing cards, unless it happened to be Christmas, and then I was choosy as to what was played.

Kenny made the announcement that they were going to draw straws. The person who drew the shortest one would be able to leave first, and so on. It seemed everyone accepted the situation. Kenny was not a person many argued with, at least if they were wise.

How exciting, I thought sarcastically. *I only hope I draw the shortest straw.*

Mike and Kenny went into the kitchen, no doubt to cut up the straws. Then Kenny came strutting out with his hand inside a brown paper bag. He came over to me first. "Pick a straw," he grunted, pushing the bag towards me. "Here, one of these I am holding between my fingers." He very cleverly worked it so that I was unable to ferret around for a short straw. I bit my tongue and pulled. I was not impressed. If I didn't have the longest straw, I must have been very close.

Around the room he went, offering the bag to each guest in turn. Finally, it became clear. I had, indeed, pulled the longest straw. *Great*, I thought, preparing for the longest night of my life.

It was a very long night. Eventually there were just two of us left, not including Mike and Kenny. Then there was just me. Finally, the host and his shadow went into the kitchen, and without waiting, I shouted a quick "Goodnight" and was on my way.

I had only a rough idea of where I was. South seemed to be the right direction, so that is the way I turned. It was almost dark, and I was way out in the country, so there were no streetlights, but the vague outline of trees were visible by the light of the quarter moon. Very soon, I came upon a gas station with a large convenience store attached. Being both hungry and thirsty, I wheeled in. The store was full of people-too full for this late at night-and although it was difficult to pinpoint just what, there seemed to be more going on than just the buying of cigarettes and bad coffee.

Having made my purchases, I proceeded to the checkout and was waiting my turn when suddenly there was a commotion. Several police cars with lights flashing and sirens screaming peeled into the parking lot, and soon the place was crawling with cops. The cashier urgently beckoned me over and told me it was a normal police raid that happened frequently at this time of night and that I ought not be involved. "You don't look like one of the people they're looking for," she reassured me. I took that as a compliment. She assisted me in a very hurried manner and rushed me out of the store. I was not sure what was going on, but it occurred to me that she seemed extremely relieved to get me out of there.

I had no idea how I would get back to the hospital, but then as I was wheeling down the main road, still headed south, a motor-cycle-riding respiratory therapist, complete with white coat, pulled up alongside and asked if I could use a ride. I did not hesitate for a second. The therapist, whom I now saw was not Don or anyone else I recognized, pointed to his sidecar, indicating I should get in. I later learned his name was Regan. He folded up my wheelchair and loaded it, rather precariously I thought. It didn't matter. I was happy to be getting a ride.

Off we went. It was quite exhilarating. After a few miles Regan turned to me and shouted, "I have to get gas." A station appeared at a fork in the road up ahead, and he slowed down. The night was dark, and the shadowy shapes of trees could be made out at the edge of the area penetrated by the station's lights.

We stopped at one of the pumps. Regan cut the ignition, swung his leg over the bike, turned, and went over to talk to someone. In the meantime, several police officers arrived. I imagined they were looking for me, but I had no idea why. If they were, the one thing that would surely give me away was the wheelchair. In the sidecar, I would appear to be just another ambulatory person.

Just as the officers were starting to question the staff at the far pumps, a man dressed in a dark grey cape and a black Stetson, whom I was sure I recognized, came out of the trees, walked quickly by the sidecar, calmly took my folded wheelchair, and disappeared into the darkness. It was Dwayne.[44]

How great! I thought. Thanks to him, I now had nothing that could give me away.

After a few minutes, Regan returned and started to gas up. By that time, the policemen had reached our pump. They looked briefly at me and then looked harder at the motorcycle and sidecar. Much to my relief, they noticed nothing unusual and walked by in the direction of the office.

The next morning, no one expressed surprise at seeing me back in my bed. I could hear the day nurses coming on duty, so knew it must have been around seven. For some reason, it always seemed the noisiest part of the day, and I often had the thought that the nurses were having a brief party before the night staff left.

The next night was totally different. Actually, it was late afternoon when I slipped out of my room. There was only one nurse on the desk, and her back was turned. I let myself out through the double doors and, in a very relaxed frame of mind, made my way to the south entrance. I stepped out of the main building and went past a small residence, which housed some of the nurses and respiratory therapists. A little further on, there was a garden, complete with benches. It was shaded and inviting, and I could not resist. I selected the best seat, made myself comfortable, and enjoyed the warm air.

In the garden, I was able to contemplate what was happening to me. I knew I could not use most of my muscles, but was encouraged by the knowledge that new limbs were growing to replace ones that no longer functioned. For example, a second right shoulder was growing anew alongside the old one. I could adopt the new one or keep the old one. It was a tough choice because I had no way of knowing which, in the final analysis, would function better.

I must have fallen asleep because I suddenly woke up and discovered I was being fastened to the seat with a couple of stout ropes. A man I didn't recognize was hurriedly tying the last knot and muttering something like, "You will freeze tonight." He then backed away. It was too late to struggle. In a flash, he disappeared.

Now what can I do? I wondered. *Someone will surely come by before long and untie me.*

Eventually, someone did. It was not yet dark, but was starting to get quite cool when from behind the trees appeared the now-familiar figure dressed in the long grey cape and Stetson. Again Dwayne had come to my rescue!

"Let's get you untied," he said. "Who did this anyway?" Before I even had a chance to reply, he was deftly cutting the ropes.

"Someone who intended me to freeze to death overnight," I suggested. "Or at the very least, someone who thought my muscles would stop growing as the temperature dropped." Before I could say more, Dwayne had vanished. I didn't even see him go. At that point, I really started to wonder if I had imagined him. However it had happened, though, I was free to move around.

By that time, it was getting decidedly cooler, and I decided to go back to the hospital. As I passed the nurse's residence, one of my nurses named Penelope was returning from her shift. "You look cold," she remarked with a concerned look. "You had better come in, and warm up."

Once inside, I found a place close to a very inviting, but rather neglected fire, put my feet up, and closed my eyes.

How does Dwayne always manage to be at the right place at the right time? I wondered.

* * *

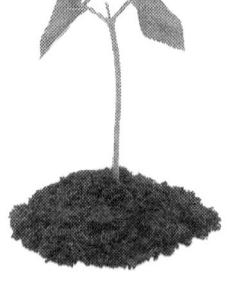

31
Sheriff's Office
...

The sun must have been pretty low in the afternoon sky because the shadow on the floor-to-ceiling window was quite clear. From my bed I could see the outline of someone wearing a cowboy hat and boots complete with spurs. The image remained stationary for a few moments and then moved away. I heard footsteps receding into the distance along a wooden sidewalk. I looked up to my headboard. Sure enough, there was my familiar drip feed, so I knew I had to be in my hospital bed, but I still wasn't quite sure.

I strained to hear whatever I could in hopes of getting a clue. Again, there were footsteps on the sidewalk. More shadows passed across the window, but nothing as recognizable as the cowboy. *This must be a western town*, I thought. *Cowboy hats, spurs, wooden sidewalks-what else could it be?*

Then, I saw the cowboy again. This time he came straight into the room and closed the door behind him. He had a gruff voice and was wearing the unmistakable star-shaped badge of a sheriff. He brushed passed my bed and went to a desk at the far end of the room, where he shuffled through some papers, walked around the desk, and then sat down. Leaning backwards in the well-padded chair, he propped up his feet, lifted the brim of his hat with a quick upward flick of his thumb, and growled at me, "So I guess they left you for us to be doing the nurse-maiding."

This was not a good start.

"I have no idea," I tried to reassure him. If this were not a good plan for him, then it certainly would not be in my best interest either. "Maybe there was an emergency at the hospital, and they needed some reliable accommodation for some of us older patients. They must trust you," I mouthed; but I don't think he could lip-read.

He took a cigar from a box on the corner of the desk and carefully cut into it with his knife. He never looked in my direction, but proceeded to light up. The sheriff-and I was now convinced he was the sheriff-was soon sitting in a swirling cloud of tobacco smoke.

At that moment, someone whom I took to be his deputy burst through the door. He appeared to be extremely agitated. "You're needed right away, boss. There's been a real bad accident behind the Main Street Bank." The two of them left in a hurry.

Why would I be left in a place like this, I wondered, *where one could be alone for hours? It may be all right for someone who isn't so dependant on others for help, but certainly not for me.* I'd no sooner formed that thought when a male nurse came into the room. As he made me comfortable, I tried to use my eyes to enquire as to why I was left here; but he didn't seem to notice and was soon on his way.

The next thing I knew it was much lighter. The sun high in the sky told me I must have slept through the night and well into the next day. I heard voices. The Sheriff and his deputy were seemingly having quite a discussion. I couldn't tell if I was the subject of their sometimes-heated debate, but I hoped not. Eventually, they put on their hats and stomped out of the office.

What now? I wondered. I was starting to get quite uncomfortable and hoped my nurse, or anyone for that matter, would come along and pay some attention to me. If only they would let me know what was happening, the waiting might not be so bad.

Some time later-it seemed like hours, but was probably only thirty minutes or so-a nurse came in and started to tidy up my bed. Soon, several others came. One was wheeling a chair. *At least I am now going to get attention, and with luck, someone will take me out of this makeshift ward.*

I was wrong.

After transferring me from the bed to the chair, all the nurses, save one, left; and I was promptly wheeled through the back door. We went through a glass door and into a sort of lobby that overlooked

Sherriff's Office

a covered walkway on the other side of which were storerooms filled with parts for beds and chairs. I didn't remember ever having been there.

The nurse parked my wheelchair, set the brake, and uttering "I'll be back in two minutes," left me on my own again. *Right*! I thought. I couldn't count the number of times I had heard that before.

People were coming and going, but no one paid more than passing attention to me. By this time, I was really confused. I couldn't have been left there to enjoy the fresh air because there wasn't any. Suddenly one of my regular nurses came in pushing an empty wheelchair.

"I see you haven't gone to sleep on me," she remarked. "That's good. I have a new chair for you to try. I'll get some help and we'll transfer you."

"Great!" I exclaimed. "Tell me though, will you then take me back to my room? I feel isolated here, and certainly don't want to be left in the Sheriff's office again."

The nurse looked at me rather oddly and then a little smile crossed her face. "The sheriff's office," she said. "What do you mean? You haven't left your room since last week!"

* * *

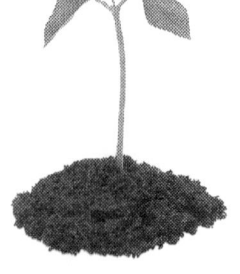

32
Ottawa Summers

I have no idea where this came from, but I was absolutely certain that every summer for the last few years, my wife and I had rented the Prime Minister's Ottawa home for two weeks of our vacation. Now we were going back, and this year, we decided to drive instead of flying.

We arrived just in time to enjoy a beautiful sunset. As expected, we had the place to ourselves. There was a note of welcome on the table in the entrance hall, telling us which rooms were open to us; how to set the security system, which had been changed from the previous year; and giving other general information.

The arrangement was perfect. We got a free vacation, and the Prime Minister was able to vacation elsewhere, secure in the knowledge that his home was cared for.

Settling in the first night was always interesting because remembering where everything was kept was a challenge. A lot could change in a year. When we'd found a home for all our belongings, we made ourselves a light meal. It had been a long day. I had done a lot of driving, and we'd found the change of air to be intoxicating. Those factors conspired to make us very tired, and we decided to turn in early. I followed the instructions about how to set the security system, and we went to bed.

It was a little like being in a high quality hotel. Our room was sumptuously decorated and had drapes of rich forest green velvet. The carpet was thick and lush. Through the large window we could look down on the well-lit courtyard. I could imagine the clip clopping of hooves on the cobblestones in the time before automobiles.

··· *A First Step* ···

It took no effort at all to fall asleep. Suddenly, however, I was wide-awake and conscious of a clamour close by. Sylvia was already out of bed and putting on her housecoat. She opened the drapes about half way and called to me. I could see flashing lights. *What on earth was happening?* I wondered?

"Brian, the courtyard is flooded! There's a fire truck, pump trucks, and even the police are here." I joined her at the window just in time to see firemen turning off water sprinklers that had obviously been running for a long time. The lawns were higher than the courtyard, which was full of water.

Who had left the sprinklers on? I considered the possibility that somehow I'd punched a wrong key on the control panel when setting the security system, but that seemed unlikely. I was sure I'd followed the instructions correctly. Maybe the head gardener or one of his people, had turned the water on and forgotten it. Whatever the cause, the damage had been done, and there was nothing we could do.

After about an hour, the activity outside settled down, and eventually, there were no more flashing lights. The flooded area must have been cleaned up. Thankfully we were not disturbed. The clean-up crew probably thought the house was unoccupied.

When we awoke the next morning, it was to the sound of heavy rain. That gave us chance to look around the house and make ourselves comfortable. The view from the lounge was exceptional. The grounds were extensive, and there were some beautiful trees, many of which I knew didn't grow in our province. We decided we were really going to enjoy this holiday.

The following day dawned under a clear blue sky. Not the day to be staying in bed, we showered, dressed, enjoyed an early breakfast, and set off on a walk through the grounds and adjoining woods. We must have gone eight or nine miles. It was almost lunchtime when we returned, just in time to see a car entering the courtyard. The driver parked and waited. He appeared to be talking to a female passenger. We went into the house, deciding that whoever it was would ring the doorbell. In the meantime, we had earned a rest and some refreshment, and that was taking priority.

A short while after we'd finished eating lunch, the bell rang. I opened the door to a man and a woman. The fellow introduced himself as Jim and told me his wife's name was Sophie. They claimed to be relatives of the prime minister and explained that the residence had been offered to them for their sole use for the next week. I shook my head in disbelief. "My wife and I rent this residence for the same two weeks every year," I said. "There has to be some mistake. Do you have anything in writing?"

"No," Sophie claimed rather indignantly, "we are family. We don't need arrangements like this in writing."

"I think you do," I said. "We have a legal lease. On your own admission, you do not. So, how can I help you?" Realizing they were at a distinct disadvantage, Sophie backed down and became more reasonable.

"This is a large residence," she said. "Couldn't we just agree to share it for a week? Perhaps you would allow us to use the west wing?"

"Come on in," I said. "We can talk about it."

After some discussion, we came to an agreement. Sylvia and I certainly had no need of the whole house, so allowing Jim and Sophie to occupy the west wing was no hardship, except that we would have to share the lounge. Since we were expecting to be out most of the time anyway, I couldn't see that it would be a problem. The next few days passed uneventfully- that is, until the third evening.

Sylvia and I had finished supper and retired to the lounge with coffee when Sophie walked in, sat herself down, and casually asked, "Could I have a coffee? My husband has decided to make an early night of it."

"Help yourself," said Sylvia. It's in the kitchen."

That was obviously not the response she wanted, and without further comment, she stomped out of the room.

I grinned at Sylvia. "Perhaps you should have prepared her supper, too," I said, ducking just in time to avoid one of her playful backhands.

The next day, after a pleasant time spent exploring our surroundings further, we decided to go out for supper. In spite of its challenging location on the twelfth floor, we chose a popular downtown restaurant, which was recognized for its excellent cuisine.

A First Step

After parking in the underground garage, we took the elevator, which for some reason, didn't go any higher than the eleventh floor. We got out and followed the signs pointing the way to the twelfth floor and eventually reached a door that appeared to open to the outside of the building, allowing a panoramic view of downtown. My first reaction was to take a step back.

When we looked past the breath-taking beauty of the sparkling city lights, we saw that beyond the door there was little more than a metal landing and a narrow stairway with short treads, much like a fire escape. The only support was a very flimsy looking rail. Neither Sylvia nor I cared much for heights. We looked at each other and, without speaking, agreed that we had to overcome this scary obstacle.

As we gingerly climbed the stairs, we tried to avoid looking down. We must have been some two hundred feet above the roadway, for vehicles looked like toys and people like ants. One glance and my stomach was in my mouth. The wind at that height was quite strong, and I had a couple of bad moments. It was with much relief that we stepped onto the upper landing only to confront outward-opening doors. Stepping backwards on a small, open landing was not my idea of fun, but we'd come this far, and it was the only way in. Amazingly, we managed to keep our balance.

Our meal was excellent and exceptionally well served. We enjoyed it, in spite of the thought of having to return down the rickety staircase when we had finished.

I paid the bill and was holding Sylvia's coat for her, when I noticed the smile on the coat check girl's face. "You won't need that, sir," she remarked, pointing to the coat.

"Why not," I asked. "It's a cool night out there, and my wife will feel the chill on her way down those outside stairs."

"No, no, no. You don't go out that way!" she exclaimed. "It's only how you come in. For leaving, we have a small elevator."

We were quite relieved. That outside staircase was treacherous, and I didn't even want to think about it.

Over the next few days we continued hiking and enjoying the countryside. The warm, sunny days made us wish we could stay an extra week. That was not to be, however, and with the holiday over, it was time to load up the car and make our way home. Little did we know what terrifying experiences lay ahead, but that's another story.[45]

* * *

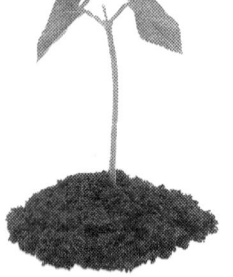

33
Quicksand Floor

My bed was going to be moved with me in it. That was a little scary. Whenever it was my turn to be moved, it was usual for me to be left-read that abandoned-in the 'halfway ward' with the unstable floor. I think there was only one such ward, and it overlooked the reservoir. From its window, you could see Woodson's Department Store, which was next to the hospital.

Sure enough, that is exactly where I was left. The nurse uttered the official mantra, "I will be back in two minutes," and continued on her merry way. Two minutes passed, then three, four, five minutes, and I was still alone. Fifteen minutes passed and still no sign of the nurse. Everything was all right for a while, but then I noticed the top of the bed appeared to be sinking. My head was lower than my feet. I peered over the edge of the bed and, to my dismay, saw that the upper end of it was most definitely sinking. Although, for the moment, the bottom still seemed on firm ground, I was terrified of being slowly swallowed up by the heaving, bubbling floor. It was as if my bed were standing in quick sand.

Where was everyone? No one had passed by since I'd been there, and there was no sign of my nurse. This was starting to feel serious. Then, just as the bed had sunk to a dangerous list, along came a nurse, who saw my predicament and rushed over. Two people, one a male nurse, responded to her pleas for help. They struggled mightily to lift the bed legs out of the floor, but with no result. The load had to be lightened; so together they lifted me off the bed and deposited me in a wheelchair in the corner.

To me, this was tremendously upsetting, although the nurses

A First Step

seemed to be taking it in stride. They retrieved the bed and moved it clear of the sinking floor. The male nurse asked me if I were all right and, without waiting for an answer, told me he would put a call out for my nurse, who should be back soon. With that, all three left the room, leaving me in the wheelchair.

It wasn't more than a couple of minutes before the floor around me again started to churn and heave. The spot under the right wheel of my wheelchair started to give way under my weight, and it wasn't long before the chair, with me in it, developed an ominous tilt. Since I couldn't use my arms, moving away was not an option. I was terrified.

"Nu-u-u-u-rse," I called as loudly as I could, "nu-u-u-u-rse, please!" Nothing happened. There was no response. Meanwhile, I was sinking deeper. The right wheel of my chair was already buried up to the axle, and the other one was now sinking, as well. I felt justified in panicking! I called out again, even louder than before.

Just when I had given up hope of anyone responding, in walked my regular nurse. She took one look at me huddled in my half-buried wheelchair and stepped back in horror. Then she pulled herself together and called for help. Another nurse came in immediately, and together they tugged at my chair until finally the wheels broke free of the floor's grip.

Another four nurses were rounded up, and the six of them transferred me back into the bed.

"Don't leave me here," I pleaded. "Park me anywhere else, but don't leave me here!" I breathed a sigh of relief as my original nurse took hold of the foot of the bed and we were on our way. We no sooner reached the doorway, however, when a 'code blue' was announced over the intercom. My nurse quickly pushed me into another room, where I found myself amongst wing chairs, sofas, and love seats. This room was obviously part of Woodson's Furniture Store. *Not again*, I thought, as once again I found myself alone.

The trouble with the code system is that the patient being left for another whose needs are desperately urgent, never knows how long he will have to wait before someone comes back for him.

Although I saw nary a nurse, I could hear members of Woodson's staff passing by the storeroom where I'd been left. As time passed, my fear of being alone returned. It was a concern that was never very far away, but on this occasion, it was acute. It got more so, as I suddenly realized how very quiet it had gotten. Now, I felt sure I had been forgotten. Although I couldn't know for certain, I thought the code blue must have either been cancelled or completed. It had been a long time, and still no one had come. Finally I heard a key turn. My heart soared, then sank just as fast. The door to my room was not being opened. It was being locked! I just knew I had been forgotten.

I had to do something. Though I felt a little groggy, I struggled out of the bed and made my way to the only window. With great difficulty, I managed to slide it open just enough to squeeze through. I dropped to the ground and found myself in the hospital's parking lot. I proceeded painfully towards a white Mobile Emergency Respiratory Assistance truck. Blessedly, it wasn't locked, and I climbed into the cab to find the keys had carelessly been left in the ignition. I gave just a moment's thought to driving away, to going home for the first time in ages, but decided I should wait for the driver and try to persuade him to take me. I desperately hoped it would be one of the guys that I knew.

Not knowing how long I would have to wait, I lay across the seat and tried to relax. The driver was not long coming. Not only wasn't he a friend of mine, but when he saw me, he became pretty belligerent.

"Caught you!" he exclaimed as if I were a vagrant. "You were just about to steal my truck, right?"

I tried to collect my composure. I was sure this driver must have been employed by 'the competition' (one of the other hospitals). I knew I was in deep trouble when my protest fell on deaf ears. His mind was obviously made up, and nothing I could say was going to change that. "I could call the police," he said, "but that would take time I don't have. I have a busy night, so I am taking you home with me until I decide what to do with you." I was in no condition to argue and imagined I would be better off to quietly comply, at least for the time being.

About twenty minutes later, we pulled into his driveway. Two children ran out to meet him followed by a woman I presumed was his wife. After shooting me an angry look, he swung out of the truck, slamming the door behind him. He then got into a heated conversation with the lady, pointing occasionally in my direction. When Don, as I heard her call him, returned to the truck, he told me, "We are transferring you to the chesterfield in our family room. You will have to stay there until I get home later tonight. Then we will figure out what we are going to do with you."

At least, I now had the prospect of being reasonably comfortable for the next few hours. The children were eyeing me with curiosity as they ran in and out of the room in play. Time passed. There were few other distractions. There was a television, but it was hidden from my view by a room divider. After what seemed like two hours or so, Don's wife came in. To my utter amazement, she started to sprinkle two-inch nails onto the unoccupied part of the chesterfield. I took this as a hostile act. I no longer had any illusions. I was in enemy territory.

For the rest of the evening, I was left pretty well to myself. I certainly felt threatened, but more than that, I was frustrated. Physically unable to get up and out of there, I had no alternative but to await the return of the 'master'. It was, perhaps, the longest evening I have ever spent.

Finally, around eleven Don returned. I could hear voices coming from the direction of the kitchen; then both he and his wife appeared at the doorway. "We are on duty tonight. We both have to go, so we are going to take you and drop you off at your place," Don asserted. With that, they helped me up from the chesterfield and carried me, somewhat clumsily, to the truck, where, after much pushing and shoving, they place me on the bunk over the driver's cab. I lay there while they packed their belongings, got on board, and drove away.

I found the truck's movement very calming-so much so, I must have been asleep within minutes. How long I slept, I don't know, but when I awoke I was in the familiar surroundings of Intensive Care, and a nurse's aide was offering me a warm blanket. I remembered nothing of how I got back there, and everyone acted as though I had never left the place; so I said nothing.

...

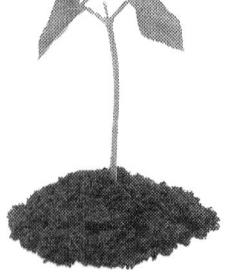

34
Precious Stone

Now, on top of everything else, I had cancer, or so I was told. I surmised, however, that I did not have to worry, because the malignancy I had was in the form of a very rare stone or crystal. I think it was in my bladder, but no one seemed too sure. This particular specimen, though, was very rare, and scientists needed a sample to keep for posterity.

Without wasting much time, I was duly prepared to travel to an army hospital in the bush. Some of the world's best scientists were either based there or associated in some way with the military establishment. My preparations included getting a shave, having my sheets changed, and having my hospital bed wheeled out and parked in the corridor. That was it. After half an hour or so, porters came and proceeded to wheel me out of the hospital. We continued across the grounds, and proceeded to the point where the main road entered the jungle. Then they just left me.

After another long wait, a great cloud of dust rose up from the dirt road. A military convoy was approaching, and it halted alongside me. I was rather unceremoniously loaded, and off we went.

Some time later, I awoke to see a white-coated doctor and a nurse holding up a jar containing their prize. It appeared to be quite a gemstone. "We discovered this rare cancer stone in your bladder," the doctor exclaimed. "Thought you might like to see it! Quite something isn't it?

"Anyway," he went on, "We have you all stitched up again, and you're quite clear. We'll have you back to Intensive Care in your own hospital tomorrow after you've had a good sleep."

··· *A First Step* ···

I should have billed them for the gemstone, I thought. Then: *What happened to the promise to get me back?* I was again on the dirt road where I had been picked up by the convoy. Although it was not getting dark yet, large crowds were congregating. My wife appeared through the crowd and joined me.

What is going on? I asked her. There were so many people around, and the crowd kept growing.

"Look at the images that are appearing," she answered, pointing to the western sky. "It's like a huge canvas of a moving pictures."

I was in awe at the wonderful sight. Imagine being in an open-air theatre with the sky as the stage and the clouds performing an absolute spectacle. It was sublime. Then, suddenly the weather changed. First the wind kicked up, eradicating the calm, and before long, the beautiful sky scenes were disappearing behind huge clouds of dust. The wind kept increasing in strength until the air was so dense with fine sandy particles that it was impossible to see. Everything that wasn't anchored down was being tossed around like so many pieces of paper. I covered my head with the bedclothes to keep from choking.

When the wind subsided a little, I peered out and saw that order was gradually appearing out of the chaos. But where was Sylvia? I looked around, but she was nowhere to be seen. Behind me was a large tented area, which I was sure hadn't been there before the storm. Or had it? *It could have been*, I reasoned, for we were, after all, quite close to the city.

Through one of the openings, I could look into the tent and see an enquiry desk, which I thought might be a good place to start looking for my wife. A kindly looking young fellow was passing, and I called to him and asked if he would mind pulling me over to the tent. He readily agreed, and once there, I was politely told by one of the staffers that I had to wait my turn. After some time, a matronly woman came over to me and asked how she could help. I asked if anyone had been looking for me, or if anyone had seen my wife. Apparently they had not. I was beginning to get a little alarmed. Not only had no one had seen Sylvia, but there was no transportation in sight to get me back to the hospital.

··· *Precious Stone* ···

Another staff member came along and suggested I was in the way and should be moved. Without waiting for a response, he pushed me into a dingy looking building on the other side of the tented area. "We will let you know when anyone enquires for you," he promised as he left me to my own devices. I found myself in a small room, furnished with only a single bed and a cane table. It was hardly the Ritz. *Let me get out of here*, I thought. *But to where? I have no way of getting to the hospital or to a decent hotel.* I didn't have any money; I had just had an operation; and I was tired. With these thoughts going through my head, I fell asleep.

It must have been several hours later when I felt someone pulling at my shoulder. It was totally dark outside. "You mustn't miss the bazaar. I'll have you transferred to a chair and wheel you around. You have to spend something or you cannot stay. " These words were muttered into my ear before I had even turned around to see who was there.

"Look," I tried to say; but I couldn't speak. *How can I let this guy know I have just had an operation?* I wondered. I couldn't even turn over to see who was addressing me.

At that moment I heard Sylvia's voice. She had Ruth with her, and they had obviously tracked me down, thankfully, just in time to help. They explained my predicament to the guy, who then pressed a small package into my hands. For some reason, I presumed it contained various good luck charms. There was a snag, though. Once the charms were accepted, the recipient was required to do favours for a group of what I believed to be religious fanatics. What those favours might be was anyone's guess, but they could be requested at any time. The sinister aspect was, the man explained, that ill fortune would befall me if I refused the charms.

Ruth suggested I raise my eyebrows once if I wished to accept the gift. I didn't hesitate. I raised my eyebrows twice.

Neither Ruth nor Sylvia approved of my choice. They were concerned about the possible implications. I was not about to be intimidated, though, and kept my hand open for the guy to take his lucky charms back. To my utter amazement, he reached for the small plastic container, tore it open, threw the contents on my bed, and stormed out.

I was destined to find small, cheap, prickly little souvenirs of that event in my bed for weeks to come. There were no precious stones, though.

My visitors, who had timed their arrival perfectly, were now offering to wheel my bed back to the hospital. I considered myself lucky. This was one of the few times I was actually looking forward to going back.

⁂

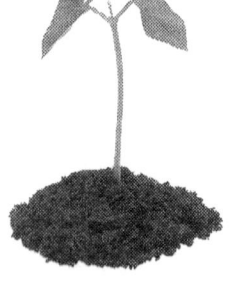

35
Underground Canal

...

My Wife, Sylvia, and I had just finished shopping in the department stores near the hospital. There was Woodson's at one end and a Wheaton's at the other. There was also a parking lot called the 'Beach Car Park', which was, as its name implied, right on the ocean. The shore there was extremely rocky, and it was common to see the breakers crashing against the rocks, sending spray in many directions. On rougher days, the spray even reached the lot, leaving a salty residue on the cars.

To the side of the lot there was a shallow cave leading to a miniature inland waterway, which although naturally formed, appeared more like an underground canal. The waterway led some four hundred yards through a rocky outcropping to another parking area, well inland.

Our car was in the inland lot, and it was getting late. 'The Beach' had been closed for an hour already, but that is where we found ourselves when we exited the store. Too late, I recalled that the only way to the inland lot from that point was through the underground canal-that is unless one had a boat in which to travel by way of the ocean. We had no boat.

Traveling on a tug in the underground canal was not without it's hazards. First, only one passenger could go at a time; second there was no crew, and the only source of power was the flow of the water; and third, the headroom in the underground tunnel was minimal, so one had to lie down, not only to avoid injury, but also to allow for forward travel. An attendant was sometimes, but not always, on hand at one end of the tunnel to give assistance.

A First Step

There was no question but that Sylvia had to go first. Reminding her to keep her head down, I helped her onto the tug, suggested she wait for me at the other end, and assured her I would see her later. I was about to push the boat off into the current when we heard a voice from just inside the tunnel.

"Hold it," I said. "It sounds like someone is stuck in there. We should check this out before you get stuck, too. Let me help you off." I reached out to assist her.

Luckily for me, there was a good length of rope on the jetty. I got into the tug, tied the rope on securely, and gave the other end to Sylvia.

"I will drift down to where the voice is and see what I can do from there," I told her. "When I give the rope a tug, that will be the signal for you to yank me back out of there."

As the current pulled me into the tunnel, the distressed voice became clearer. It was obviously a woman. It was difficult to see in the darkness, so I raised myself up as much as I dared and reached out in case I bumped into something. My arm was pushed aside and almost trapped as I brushed against the other boat. Holding tight, I managed to stop and told the woman to keep calm and I would try to get her out of there.

Per my arrangement with Sylvia, I tugged on the rope. Slowly the two boats responded to her pulling. I could visualize what an effort it must have been. Slowly, inch-by-inch, we moved against the flow. After anxious minutes, we were back at the Beach Car Park. Sylvia, it seemed, had saved the day. Now we could pay attention to the unfortunate lady, who had a big gash across her forehead.

"What happened?" I asked, "Did you sit up in the tunnel?"

"Yes," she replied. "The boat got wedged against something, and as I was raising myself up to see how to get free, it lurched forward. I didn't get my head down quickly enough."

"You go through again with Sylvia following right behind," I suggested, glancing at my wife for her agreement. "You must have your injury attended to, and that cannot happen here."

I helped the women into their respective tugs, pushed them off, and proceeded to follow. For some reason my boat moved really slowly, and by the time I arrived at the inland car lot, there was no sign of anyone. *Sylvia must have wasted no time in getting the injured lady to a clinic*, I decided.

I made my way to the second floor of the lot where I thought I had left our car. When it wasn't there, I checked the other levels, but it was nowhere to be seen. I finally found it in a dark corner on the ground level. With relief, I went towards it, feeling in my pocket for the keys. When I got close to the car, I could see a fairly large cardboard sign leaning against it. The message read: "Don't drive this car. You are too handicapped and will be a danger to everyone else on the road. The police have been informed and will be watching."

I thought I knew whose work this was, but couldn't be sure. Whoever it was, they were right, of course. I decided right then and there that I would leave the car and walk.

As I headed home, it was starting to get dark. I had not gone far, when a white RTSV pulled up alongside, and the driver, whom I recognized, but whose name escaped me, offered me a ride, which I gladly accepted.[46]

"Can you drop me off at home?" I asked.

"You should be back at the hospital, shouldn't you?"

"I guess so, but they are not doing anything with me, so I might as well be at home. No one misses me, although I assume they are keeping a record of my attendance." I noted the smile that crossed his face as I spoke. "By the way," I continued, "I'm embarrassed to say I have forgotten your name."

"Alan," he replied. "I'm not surprised you can't remember. I only saw you a couple of times when you first came in, and it's been a while. Anyway, I have to make a couple of calls; then I've been invited out for drinks. Would you like to join us? I think you will know some of the others at the party."

"I don't see why not," I replied, thinking I really didn't have much choice.

"Then why don't you make yourself comfortable in the back? If you fall asleep, I'll wake you when we get to Marty's. That's where the party is."

Thanking him, I made my way to the back of the truck, grabbed a couple of pillows, and proceeded to stretch out on one of the bench-

A First Step

es. I noticed these vehicles were well equipped and were built to the same specifications as those intended for flight. The only difference was that the latter had wings made of two-by-fours and had a dismal safety record.

The next thing I knew, Alan was gently shaking my shoulder. At least I thought it was Alan. As things turned out, it was someone rather more attractive. She was holding my hand, searching for a vein, and offering to take some blood. I was no longer in the back of the truck!

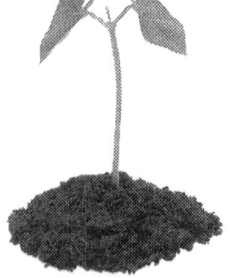

36
Heavy Snowfall Warning

Here I was downtown, but in my hospital bed with my oxygen and intravenous feeding equipment hanging from the headboard. It was four in the afternoon, and I was hoping to get a lift back to the hospital. The traveling respiratory therapists (RT's) had arranged to meet me at the corner of Fourth and Fourth, where I had just arrived. It was starting to snow. To pass some time, I traveled farther down the block to Radio Hut and spent a little time window shopping and watching a show on their large-screen TV.

I was about to leave when the program changed and a heavy snowfall warning flashed across the screen. The programming then returned to normal, but I realized I did not know which areas were affected by the warning or even if my city, Calgary, was included, so I decided to stay a little longer, hoping for a repeat. I didn't have to wait long. Yes, the warning was intended for Calgary, so I now paid a lot more attention. It seemed very serious. Commuters and others in the downtown area were advised not to leave, but to find accommodation wherever they found themselves. At least 25 CM. of snow were expected, along with extremely high winds. That spelt blizzard conditions.

Just my luck! I thought. *How could I arrange accommodations that would be accessible in my hospital bed?* I decided to make my way back to the corner of Fourth and Fourth in hopes that my RT friends would show up. By now it was snowing heavily, and my pillows and blankets were getting covered, so to stay dry, I had to keep my head well down under the covers. *This is no good*, I thought. *I had better try to make for Woodson's and get some shelter.*

··· *A First Step* ···

I can't remember where I parked my bed, but I do remember being on a shuttle bus looking over the driver's shoulder and seeing what was perhaps the worst winter weather I had ever witnessed. It was a complete whiteout. The snow was falling so heavily, it was virtually impossible to see anything. After we had gone a few blocks, the driver turned to me and asked which of Woodson's entrances I needed. I marvelled at the fact that he could identify a particular entrance through the blinding snow.

"It doesn't matter," I responded. "Just drop me where you can."

Once inside store, I made my way to the central escalator and proceeded to the top floor. As I reached the third floor, I was pleasantly surprised to see Ken Waterton, one of my colleagues from the office. It was natural that the weather would be the first topic of conversation.

"If this continues, I guess we are both here for the night," I commented. There was no sign of it abating.

"I think you're right. Have you ever used the Woodson Club when you were stuck downtown overnight?" he asked.

I was rather confused by the question and said quite truthfully that I had not. I didn't even know that the Woodson Club existed. I had thought I'd just make myself comfortable between a couple of counters, using my rather generously sized parka as a blanket. I liked Ken's idea better. "Okay," he said. "Why don't we go to the restaurant on the top floor, get some food, and afterwards we can go to the Club and I will introduce you. You will be more comfortable there."

"Sounds good to me," I replied.

Over supper, I quizzed him about the Woodson Club. Apparently it cost two hundred dollars to get in; but he explained that there was an outside overhead rail system, which ran from the top floor, and if we climbed onto one of the railcars at mid-floor, we could get in free.

"I don't understand, " I said. "Is there no other way in? How does this rail system work?"

"Well, there is if you want to pay $200," he explained. "The outside rail system is a one way downhill track around perimeter of the building. It serves as an alternative to elevators to reach certain floors including high security areas, and will suit us just fine.

"I know what your next question will be," he continued. You want to know how we enter the system at mid-floor? After we've had supper, I will demonstrate. It's quite easy. We do have to act quickly, though, as you will see. Basically at each mid-floor point there is a turnout from the main track, and usually a spare railcar is parked there. The trick is to apply the brakes so that the railcar coming down stops just past the turnout. We then have to reroute the track to allow the parked railcar to run downhill and connect up with the main train. This is all run by computer, so after being braked between floors, the car only stops for sixty seconds, and then automatically restarts; but it's enough time for us to hop in."

"Sounds dangerous," I said. "You do seem to be familiar with the whole operation, though. So let's say I'm game."

I wondered later how the railcars running from the top and then circling around the building down to the basement ever got back up to where they started.

After finishing supper we decided to have a couple of drinks while contemplating Ken's plan for hitching a ride on the railcar system. I asked how we could get to the rail track in between this and the lower floor. He indicated by a casual gesture that we could gain access through the fire exit door just behind us. All we had to do was make this look very innocent and not attract any attention.

"Let's go now," he said abruptly, "while there are not to many people around."

With that, we drank up and slipped through the fire exit. There was a flight of stairs, and at the halfway point there was a doorway, which we entered. Ken seemed a bit hesitant, but upon hearing railcar traffic around the next corner, he said he guessed we were headed in the right direction. Sure enough, we came upon a spare railcar just where we expected to find it. Taking my lead from Ken, I set the trackside brake, returned to the railcar, and jumped in as he went for the handbrake. Now all we had to do was wait for the next train.

We didn't have long to wait. Moments later a three-car train was

A First Step

brought to a halt by the brake we had set. By now, high winds were blowing snow over us, making the footing rather treacherous. I was very aware of the abyss below.

We had to move fast since the train was almost stopped. Ken released the brake, and I jumped out to change the turnout switch, hopping back in just in time. In the meantime, Ken had jumped out and connected our car to the main train. He was also just in time, and soon the whole train, including our car, was gaining speed. Twice, we were stopped by people joining the train the same way we had.

"Which floor are we making for Ken?"

"The second," he said. "It's the only way into the club!"

As he made his comment, we reached our destination. We were now able to mingle with the fare-paying passengers, as tickets no longer had to be shown. That made me feel a lot better.

The club entrance was nothing spectacular, just old-fashioned double swinging doors with an attendant behind a desk just inside. Ken introduced me and showed his pass, which allowed access for him and a guest. We passed through the lobby and entered a rather large hall. At this point Ken pointed to a pile of blankets and pillows in the middle of the floor and suggested that I help myself and find a spot to bed down for the night. Then he turned and left.

I saw one or two people I recognized from the hospital, and they acknowledged me as I went by. I grabbed some blankets and looked for a place to settle in. Many people had obviously arrived earlier than Ken and I, so space was at a premium. I noticed that most had paired off and had a momentary pang about being alone.

On finding a gap, I bedded down and prepared to go to sleep for the night feeling thankful that I had shelter and wasn't stranded outside in the blizzard. Just as I was about to doze off, who should walk through the door but Clarisa, one of my nurses! She recognized me immediately and waved. I couldn't help feeling flattered. She was a very caring nurse and a very attractive young lady.

I didn't expect that Clarisa and her companion-whom I thought I recognized as another nurse-would want to talk to me. She appeared to know some of the people and chatted with several acquaintances as she made her way to a group in the far corner. After what seemed to be a brief conversation, though, Clarisa left the group and came in my direction.

"Hi Brian," she greeted me, "could I ask you a favour?"

"Of course." I replied. "How can I help?"

"I'm not sure that I'm too comfortable here. The group in the corner is expecting me to stay with them, and quite frankly, I don't wish to. Can I tell them that you have invited me to share your blanket?"

"Sure, no problem."

With that, she placed her drawstring bag down beside my pillow, thanked me, and said she would be back in a few minutes. Ironically, 'Back in a few minutes' is what all the nurses say all the time!

True to her word, this time, she in fact was back in a few minutes. Her nursing instincts appeared to take over, and she asked how my feet were. Any Guillain-Barré patient will appreciate the importance of that enquiry, because if the feet are comfortable, it is likely that the patient is comfortable, overall.

"They're sort of okay." I replied. "They do have a restless feeling though."

Clarisa responded by uncovering my feet and giving them a gentle massage. Anything less than gentle could prove extremely painful.

After a short time, she finished her massage, took off her shoes and street clothes, and went to the blanket storage area in the middle of the hall for a thicker blanket. She was concerned that I was sleeping directly on the floor. After rolling me over on my side and sliding the new blanket under me, she returned me to my original position and then felt my forehead as though to check out my temperature, and continued stroking my brow.

I was always putty in the hands of anyone who ran fingers through my hair or did anything pleasant to my head. I even loved having my hair washed or getting a haircut. I found Clarisa's touch very soothing.

All good things come to an end, however, and after a while she stood back and said, "It's bedtime, Brian." With that, she reached across for the edge of my blanket and slipped under it. After giving me a hug, she turned her back to me, snuggled up close, pulled my arms around her, and that's how we went to sleep.

After a couple of hours, I awoke, tried to rise up on my elbows, intending to gently kiss Clarisa's cheek, but could not. She must have awoken at the same time and realized what I was trying to do because she raised her cheek towards me, accepting my gesture. Then we slept again, and that is all I remember.

The next morning I found myself in my hospital bed in the same intensive care room that I had occupied for some time. Sure enough, I could hear the regular 'clip clop, clip clop' of my ventilator, and I gained comfort from that and the sight of my intravenous drip-feed equipment. I didn't have to worry about the retrieval of my hospital bed parked somewhere downtown...probably covered with two feet of snow!

But wait! I thought to myself. *If my hospital bed is still parked somewhere downtown, whose bed am I in now? And how on earth did I get back here?*

...

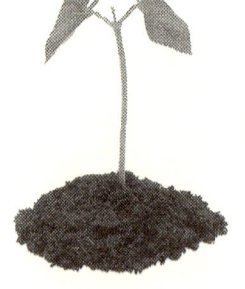

37
Downtown Adventures

Somehow I made it downtown again, and into the Plus Fifteen system.[47] It was getting rather late and was time to start looking for some accommodation. As it turned out, I didn't have very far to go.

I think it was somewhere near 9th Avenue that I saw a small hotel just off the Plus Fifteen. *That should be worth exploring*, I remember thinking. *I could be independent for once and avoid going back to the hospital.* I liked what I saw. It didn't look very expensive and appeared to offer suitable accommodations, so I booked in for later that evening and took some time to wander around.

The first stop was to be the bank, as I needed money. On the way, I heard what was becoming a very familiar sound. I was on one of the many bridges that criss-cross the downtown area. It had a stairwell that went to the roadway below, and I heard several cars using their new musical horns.[48] It wasn't an unpleasant sound, although it could get annoying after a while. Actually, it made me feel as though I were on vacation in some other part of the world. Europe, perhaps.

Unfortunately, by the time I reached the bank it was closed. Now I had a problem.

With no cash, I was stuck. Sure I had a wallet full of plastic, but being unable to use my hands, I could not sign a receipt. I tried to think of a way around it. I had already booked my hotel room and given the clerk my credit card number, so perhaps I could arrange for my wife to meet me in the morning, and she could sign. It was worth a try.

I wandered around for a while longer and then decided to call it a night. I went back to the hotel, but to my surprise, things were a little different than they had been earlier in the day. For one thing, a whole area opposite the check-in counter had been opened up, revealing a number of single beds and a couple of washrooms with padlocks on the doors. *Wait a minute*, I thought. *I hope they are not going to give me one of those beds.*

Turning to the busy reception area, I signalled to one of the clerks and was politely asked to wait. I spent the next few minutes anxiously tapping out a rhythm on the counter. I feared the worst. There was a convention in the city, and it was soon obvious from the replies others were receiving that rooms were at a premium.

When my turn came, I asked the clerk for my room key. He turned to the board, then, as though suddenly remembering something, he turned back to face me saying he was sorry, but I had been allocated one of the beds opposite the desk. "The rest of the hotel is fully booked," he explained, and seeing the look of amazement on my face, added, "There is not a room left anywhere in the city."

"But, there is no privacy in that area," I insisted.

"We have a screen that can be drawn across to separate that space from the reception area, and I will have that arranged immediately, sir."

I complained one more time, though I knew I would get nowhere.

"Sorry, sir. If we could do better, we would," was the only response I would get. He pointed to the bed allocated to me.

So it is either this or nothing, I thought.

"All right, I will take it," I said, Then I spun my chair around, wheeled into the area temporarily set aside for bedrooms, and dumped my belongings on the bed earmarked for me. I knew it would be too late to arrange for transportation to anywhere else. Somehow I made it under the covers and was able to fall asleep, but not before two thoughts crossed my mind. The first was *I wonder if the hospital staff will miss me tonight?* The second was *Why have they put padlocks on the washroom doors?*

I was soon to have the answer to that second question. I was awakened many times during the night by people coming and going, and much of the traffic seemed to consist of non-residents. Then there were the late night revellers using their musical car horns on the street below. A small window just above my bed opened up to what I guessed to be 10th Avenue. I finally decided further sleep was out of the question, so I had lots of time to worry about paying the hotel bill.

I planned to climb out of bed before anyone stirred. I would quietly get my belongings together and slip out of the main door without being seen. They would have my credit card number, so I hoped they would not accuse me of leaving without paying the bill. I would ask my wife to stop by later in the day and sign to settle the account.

It was a great plan in theory, but in spite of everything, I must have fallen asleep again. When I woke up, there was a bustle of activity and the sun was high in the sky. I clearly had to change my plan. I would have to talk my way out of this situation. Then something quite unexpected happened. Someone was tugging at my arm.

"I am having difficulty locating your vein," I heard the white-coated woman say. "I am going to leave this to the doctor."

On looking around it was soon obvious that I was in my bed in Intensive Care. So I had not managed to avoid going back to the hospital, after all.

The next night was different. This time I really was going downtown. I made it in my traveling bedstead to the mezzanine in one of the centrally located office towers. Luckily, I had help getting on and off a public elevator, into which my bed fit with only an inch to spare; otherwise I wouldn't have made it to the second floor. The occasion was an exhibition, which I did not want to miss. I ran into a number of people I knew and could spend time talking to.

The evening passed quickly, and it was soon time to leave. I was just about to call it a day, when I spotted one of my nurses, Betsy. She looked most surprised to see me there.

"Brian, you should not be out of the hospital!" she exclaimed.

"Why not?" I asked. Nothing is happening there, and I am never missed. And there is so much to do here." Then as an afterthought: "Are you going back there now?"

"No," she said. I am one of the organizers and expect to be here until well after midnight."

··· A First Step ···

We talked for quite a while. Finally she excused herself to get some work done, and I decided to leave. A janitor came to my rescue and pushed my bed towards the elevators. As we got closer, he paused, and reminded me that the public elevators were closed for the night. Scratching his head, he wondered out loud how I could exit the building. He eventually decided he would have to leave me where I was and seek help.

I waited for quite a while. In the end, Betsy came across me again and, upon realizing my predicament, offered to help. She remembered there was a service elevator in the back and thought we could use that. *Thank goodness*, I thought. It would not be much fun to be trapped in here for the night.

With the help of the janitor, we made it to the ground floor and then outside. It was cold, and I shivered as I thanked my rescuers. I hoped one of the familiar white RT trucks would soon arrive to give me a lift.

It was starting to snow very lightly, but enough so that after a few minutes my bed was covered. Fortunately, it was the dry stuff, otherwise my sheets would have been soaking wet. Thankfully, I did not have long to wait. The RT truck driver must have spotted me from over half a block away, as he very smoothly changed lanes and pulled up just ahead of me. "Look," he said, "I can't take you straight back because I'm on my way to a party. Would you like to come with me? You will know most of the guys there. My name is Malcolm, by the way."

Without a moment's hesitation I agreed, which I think is what he expected; and he loaded me on as though this were purely routine.

We drove for about fifteen minutes, then turned into the driveway of a large mansion. "What are you doing here?" I questioned. "This is the home of the city police chief, and it is not likely he would be holding a party for us."

"Don't worry," Malcolm replied. "I believe he is out of town. It's his daughter who is throwing the party. She is one of the nurses from the hospital. You probably know her."

The front door was unlocked, so in we went. Moving through the crowd of people who were already there, we made our way to the kitchen, figuring out where it was by observing where the food was coming from. Then from somewhere behind me, I heard a familiar voice, "Hi Brian, glad you made it." I spun around to see a nurse named Clara.

"I need to sit down," I told her. She looked around and quickly came to the conclusion the safest thing would be to take me up the stairs at one side of the kitchen, which seemed to lead nowhere except to a series of upper storage cupboards. At the top was a seat, which could be unfolded from the wall.

She has to be joking, I thought hopefully. But, this was no joke. Clara, it seemed, was not above giving me a bad time. She had arranged for volunteers to assist me up the stairs, giving me little option but to do her bidding. Everyone else in the kitchen, and Clara's boyfriend in particular, area seemed highly amused at my predicament. There I was, stuck up in the air, feeling like a fool. Upon closer investigation, I realized the boyfriend looked familiar. Then it hit me that virtually every guest was an employee of our largest competitor, and they were really enjoying seeing their competition having a bad time.

Everyone except me was enjoying the party. I watched as supper was prepared in the kitchen below me. Clara was close by loading a tray of fresh fruit. I called to her over the din and asked if her father was aware of this party in his absence. She gave me a look that told me it was not a good question to ask.

What had happened, I wondered, *to make Clara so antagonistic towards me?* She was always so friendly and helpful at the hospital, but not so now. *Maybe it was boyfriend trouble or maybe her father was coming home unexpectedly.* I had no chance to converse with her, so there wasn't much hope of getting answers.

I was getting tired of being the butt of jokes in the kitchen. Also, by this time, I was really sleepy.

Finally, Malcolm, whom I had not seen since our arrival, came to the rescue. "Let's go and find you a chesterfield," he said. "There's no way we will be leaving here tonight." I was only too happy to agree.

Within half an hour, I was in a spacious lounge. I'd been bathed and placed on the owner's favourite and expensively covered chesterfield. It wasn't the best place for a patient in my condition, but I was too tired to argue.

I awoke with a start. It must have been the following afternoon. I was still on the same chesterfield, but now I was surrounded by what appeared to be family members and friends of Clara. Some were quietly talking, others were reading, and a few were knitting. Clara noticed I was awake and, with none of the previous night's antagonism, asked if I were okay. *Was the party last night just a dream?* I wondered.

Without waiting for my reply, she added, "Malcolm just phoned, and he will be here to pick you up in about an hour. It's snowing pretty hard-almost a white out-and there have been a lot of accidents. It's a pity you have to go out in this weather."

I wondered how they were going to transfer me into the truck, but I was grateful to be someplace warm and dozed off again.

Next thing I knew someone was gently shaking my arm and saying, "Wake up, wake up! It's time to get you in your chair." It was one of my nurses, and I was in my room in Intensive Care. *How did Malcolm get me back without waking me?*

"Did you just change the sheet?" I asked. "The other one must have been wet from the snow."

The nurse gave me a funny look. She must have thought I'd been dreaming!

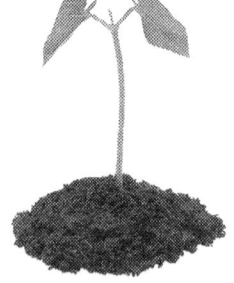

38
Part Time Patient

I couldn't decide whether I was a hospital patient or not. I knew, however, that I was overseas.

In the daytime I was able to go anywhere I wished, either by car or on foot. It was odd, since although I knew in my inner being that I was in the hospital, no one seemed to miss me. It seemed I didn't spend much time there at all.

The hospital was on an island that used to be a British Colony. There was a small city close by, and I seemed to spend a lot of time near its harbour. I also spent a great deal of time at the Harbour Cliff Hotel, which was just off the road leading to the water. I always tried to make it there for lunch, since they served up good food and were not too expensive.

The evenings were a different matter. The hotel was extremely crowded, and it was difficult to get any attention, particularly for me as I had trouble getting around. However, this evening was to be different.

I had just left the car and was crossing the road in front of the Harbour Cliff when I heard what the familiar sound of musical car horns. The sound was so distinctive that you just couldn't miss it. I turned and smiled. It reminded me of home. Just before we left, these horns were becoming very popular. Now, they were obviously being sold here.

Continuing towards the entrance, I checked in my pocket for my wallet, pushed against the revolving doors, and immediately found myself in a mass of humanity. People were milling around everywhere.

I had been here often enough to know my way around and made

straight for the lower floor, which was a favourite of the locals. It was more crowded than it had ever been before. With difficulty, I made my way to a table, sat down in the only vacant seat, and waited for the server. It was then that I spotted two women who I thought looked familiar. One of them had seen me, too and was waving in recognition.

I decided to try to join them. *Try* was the operative word, since I was having a tough time moving my legs.

Finally, after much struggling, I reached the ladies' table. Now I saw they were two of my nurses, Colette and Patricia. They made room, then proceeded to scold me for being there.

"You should not be out of the hospital," Patricia remonstrated. "Why do you do it?"

"Nothing ever happens in the day-time, and no one ever misses me, so why shouldn't I do some exploring?" I reasoned. "I can't just sit around doing nothing-but, please don't mention this to the patient-care manager or the doctors."

"Brian," Colette said with deliberate emphasis. "What are we going to do with you?" They both laughed, obviously realizing it was hopeless to try and talk me out of my exploits.

"Let me buy you a drink," I suggested, hoping it would divert them from this subject.

"How are you getting back to the hospital?" Patricia asked.

"I am not really sure," I responded. "Usually a respiratory therapist picks me up in one of their trucks. They seem to know where I will be at any given time. There is probably one waiting outside for me right now."

At that moment, Patricia's husband, Desmond, showed up. He was the designated driver, it seemed, and his arrival was the signal that it was time to leave. Colette turned to me, and suggested I go with them. "If your RT truck is waiting for you," she said with a big smile, "that's fine; but if not, you are coming with us. We are not leaving you here." I agreed. To argue would have been pointless. We made our way to the lobby and out the revolving doors.

There was no large white truck to be seen anywhere. I was disappointed. I knew my companions had not believed me, and I wanted to demonstrate that I was not imagining that the respiratory therapists provided transportation for me. Colette looked knowingly in my direction. "I don't see anyone waiting for you," she teased, as we proceeded towards Desmond's car.

Desmond helped me get in, and we were on our way to an apartment the three of them shared-because of the cost Colette later explained. I must have been lulled to sleep by the smooth ride because, the next thing I knew, we had arrived at our destination.

Once inside the very comfortable apartment, hot coffee was the order of the day. After sitting around talking enjoying the warm glow of a log fire, Desmond turned to Patricia and explained he was on an early shift the next day. "We had better take our leave of these two, and get moving," he added.

"Sure," Patricia responded. "I have an early start too. 'Night guys. See you whenever."

It was then that it dawned on me I had gone to the Harbour Cliff Hotel in my car. It was, however, too late to do anything about it, since Desmond would not appreciate having to get out of bed and run me back for it. *Oh well, I will just have to pick it up tomorrow*, I thought.

"Brian, you look miles away," Colette remarked, as she finished tidying up the room.

"Sorry," I replied, rather lamely. "You guys have been so kind. I think the warmth from the fire has gotten to me." She was making herself comfortable on the rug and gazing into the hearth. She looked very thoughtful for a moment, then turned to me and posed the question, "Are you interested in history?" She sure knew how to get my attention. History and politics were among my favourite subjects.

"Yes, indeed," I told her. "And I presume from the question that you are, also. Do you have a favourite period?"

Once on that topic of mutual interest, we covered everything from the Black Death in the Middle Ages to English Kings and Queens up to the reign of Victoria. Time passed so quickly, and it must have been well after two AM when the doorbell rang. Colette jumped up, peeked out the window and, upon recognizing the visitor, opened the door. I could tell from the guest's distinctive voice that it was Clint, the respiratory therapist.

"I am here to give Brian a ride," he said.

"How did you know he was here?" she asked.

"That was easy," he responded, smiling. "One of the other respiratory therapists saw him leaving the Harbour Cliff with you guys. We all know he's a late-nighter!"

"Well, I guess we have to call it a day," I said, turning to the good-natured Colette. "Thanks for your hospitality. I hope I haven't kept you up too late." I gripped her hand as a thank-you gesture. She responded with a gentle kiss on my cheek.

"Good night, Brian. You get yourself safely back to the hospital."

With that, Clint and I left to get into the white RT truck, and as we did, he gave me a broad grin. "Nice lady!"

...

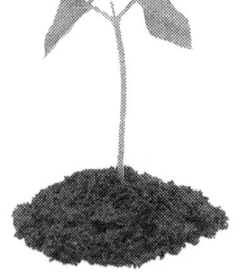

39
Daylight Robbery

For some reason, I liked to window shop in one particular small hobby and craft store, but never spent any money there. Others also must have done more looking than buying because there were notices that the store was closing down. This made me sad. I had spent many grey winter afternoons there happily browsing.

I wondered if someone else would take it over or if maybe the place would be gutted. Nothing stays the same forever.

Very soon my questions were answered. There was good news and there was bad news. The bad news was that a retired army colonel with a reputation for being unethical and taking advantage of others had announced his intention to purchase the business. The good news was that he apparently planned to continue running it as a hobby and crafts store.

One item in the store that had always fascinated me was a special sort of modelling clay. At normal room temperature, it was stiff, but when being handled warmed it up, it would become soft and pliable. It was used mainly to make scale models of finely detailed buildings, exterior fences, and walls. There were models of buildings sculpted and moulded by the staff on display.

Some time passed before I visited the shop again. When the next opportunity presented itself, I could sense many changes. For one thing, I was conscious of being under surveillance from the moment I walked in. *So, this is how the new owner is going to operate*, I thought. After a quick walk through, I decided enough was enough. It just wasn't the same store, so I left.

I couldn't keep away for long, though. I was fascinated by the pos-

A First Step

sibilities offered by that modelling clay; so a few days later, I decided to go back and buy a few dollars worth. When I arrived, I saw the new owner had raised the prices substantially; and there was also a notice warning shoppers that they would be required to purchase the product if, in handling it, they altered the shape or form of the product. As on the last visit, it was soon obvious I was under surveillance. That made me very angry and I became determined to fight back.

As I handled the clay models, I was careful not to change their shape-something that could happen just from the heat of one's hand. A large woman, whom I suspected was the store detective, watched every move I made. She appeared to be known to a number of the shoppers. Even when she stopped to talk to someone else, she kept her eyes on me. To make life difficult for her, I would turn away and, when I was done with an item, I'd put it down outside her line of sight. That would drive her crazy! This cat and mouse game continued for most of the afternoon. I was determined not to be outdone, but I think she had other ideas.

A short while later, the new owner made his entrance. He went straight over to the store detective, and the two of them went into a huddle. It didn't surprise me to see them looking and pointing from time to time in my direction. I was sure the heat would now be on me, but in what way, I could never have guessed.

It was getting near closing time when I took a last look at the clay models. I picked up a model of a bungalow and spent a little time admiring the detail inside. I was too engrossed to notice the detective crank up the heat. As it turned out, I was standing right under a duct and, all of a sudden, it was getting very warm. I loosened my collar, then became aware that the clay model I was holding was starting to get really soft, and indentations were appearing in the clay where my palm and fingers came in contact with it. The harder I tried to smooth it out, the more of a mess I made.

"That will be $175, please." A sales assistant had moved up behind me and obviously decided I'd changed the appearance of the model and would have to pay for it. "Please take it to the check-out and settle up there," she continued.

··· *Daylight Robbery* ···

What an underhanded way to get me to buy something. I decided that to sink that low, they must have been pretty desperate for income. There was no doubt the product had been changed somewhat, but that would not have happened had they not deliberately turned up the heat.

At that point, my wife came in looking for a ride home. I explained what had happened, and we were in total agreement as to how we should handle this situation. I replaced the model, turned to the sales assistant, and asked her to accompany us to the checkout. After complaining about the way I had been tricked, I assured the cashier and sales assistant that I would accept some responsibility and consider a reasonable claim, but refused to pay in full for the item I had allegedly damaged.

"Then we shall have to charge you with shoplifting," asserted the store detective, who had joined the group.

"Sorry," I responded. "Not only am I taking nothing out of the shop, I am inviting you to submit a claim, which, if reasonable, will be accepted. Here is my address. That cannot be called shoplifting by anyone's definition."

The response from the store detective was rather predictable. "The new owner would not agree," he said emphatically. "He has a very aggressive policy regarding losses of any kind; and it is my duty to implement that policy. If you don't pay up, you will be arrested the moment you leave the shop. We have already called the police." I turned to my wife and suggested we withdraw to the back of the store and discuss the situation further.

As soon as we were out of sight, we went through a doorway leading to some stairs. They led into a large storage area, where we proceeded to hide among all the packages, cartons, and supplies. On the way up I opened a window to make it appear we had made our escape that way. It must have worked because the subsequent search of the storage area was very perfunctory.

After waiting for things to settle down, we decided to climb out of the open window and make our way to the car under the cover of darkness. To our dismay, when we reached the window and leaned out to make sure the coast was clear, we saw the flashing lights of two police cars. They must have known we were still there and were waiting for us to come out. This called for a different plan. We climbed out of the window, keeping as low a profile as possible. Instead of making for the car, we went the opposite way into a wooded area and made our way through the trees to the main road. Then we walked home.

The next morning I awoke in need of a suction. The day nurse came in to check me out and promised to call a respiratory therapist. While awaiting relief, I couldn't help wondering how long it would be before the craft and hobby store filed a claim. This worried me somewhat, although I knew they would not succeed in a charge of shoplifting. Still, I was dealing with someone who was unscrupulous, so I imagined anything could happen.

Days later, my wife came in on her daily visit and held out a letter from the hobby store. It was a claim for $750! "That is outrageous," I told Sylvia. Could you reply for me? Tell them, under the circumstances, we make a counter offer of $75, which will be withdrawn if not accepted within thirty days. Even that is being more generous than they deserve."

We never heard anything further on the subject. No wonder, really. A few months later, I came to the realization there was no hobby shop or any other store in the place I had imagined it.

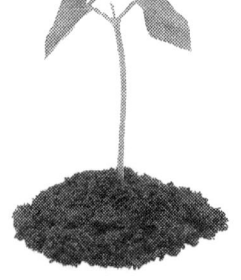

40
Neck Brace

I was convinced that the reason a neck brace was put on me every time I was transferred from my hospital bed to a wheelchair was to make me look foolish. I imagined it gave me the likeness of an English comic figure, Billy Bunter. Billy was, as I recall, a very plump and greedy fellow with ugly, fat protruding lips accentuated by sunken cheeks. That is exactly how the brace made me feel.

The brace had two parts with an opening in the front of the bottom half for connections to the ventilator or the oxygen supply. The connection had to be changed whenever I was taken farther away from the ventilator than the cable would allow. I was, naturally, more conscious of wearing it when I was out of my room, and that made me suspicious of the motives of anyone suggesting such an outing.

If it were a publicity stunt, a significant number of people must have been involved, I figured, because it took six or seven nurses to get me out of bed and into the chair. I was sure they were not all involved, though, since most of them were very kind and caring. The whole thing appeared to me to be the work of the director of the government department that was interested in publicizing and obtaining support for Guillain Barré Syndrome patients and their families, better known as the department of PS-GBS-PAF. The trouble was, I could not identify him.

I did not like anything about PS-GBS-PAF! I did not like the way they worked or their personnel.

One afternoon I recall being prepared for what was to become a familiar outing. On went my brace, and I endured a transfer to the wheelchair. I knew I was surrounded by friends, yet I was equal-

··· A First Step ···

ly sure there was at least one person from the 'department' in their midst.

It was a beautiful sunny day, and so warm and comfortable that, except for the brace, I was starting to forget about all my suspicions. Not for long though. Suddenly I was flooded with the knowledge that something was being planned for me. *I was to be enlisted on a secret mission.*[49]

※ ※ ※

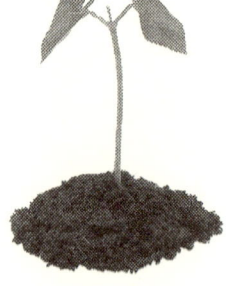

41
The Debt Collector

Someone had left a summary of the cost of my hospital stay on the notice board in my room. I could see it quite clearly from my bed and recall it being in the neighbourhood of $22,000-and that was just for the first month in the Rockyview Hospital!

Why had it been left there, I wondered? *Was it to remind me they needed my money?* Now I had something else to worry about. *Wasn't the province covering all health care costs? Did I have to come up with all this money? Surely not.*

For a time I was able to ignore the notice, feeling that if I did, the problem might go away. Several days passed and nobody referred to it. There were, of course, a number of other possibilities. Maybe the management simply wanted patients to know what the cost of their treatment and accommodation was; or maybe it was someone's idea of a joke.

My concern about the notice continued for the next few days. Then to make matters worse, a desk appeared just outside of my door, and eventually someone whom I did not recognise, sat there armed with papers and a variety of folders. She put a notice on her workstation that read, 'All accounts to be paid here'. *Now*, I asked myself, *why outside of my door? Has this been done for a reason?*

I imagined it would be possible for me to pay the costs for a month or so, but after that, it would take a serious bite out of our savings. *Perhaps if I could pay for just one month*, I reasoned, *I could stall them from throwing me out and manage to stay for one additional month.*

This problem had me worried for some time. Was it a dream, or reality?[50]

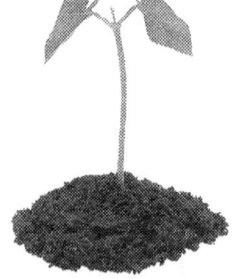

42
Flying Bombs

I had successfully persuaded my wife to join me for a day's outing to the mountains. The Rockies always provided a welcome change from city living, and we had both been working hard and were convinced we needed a short break. We were approaching Banff on Highway 1. It was almost mid-day, and we were starting to get hungry. Rounding a bend in the road, we saw a most unusual sight. At the side of the road was a huge billboard, unusual in that such advertising was not normally permitted along the highway. It was promoting a new low-cost aircraft, claiming that for fourteen thousand dollars it was possible to acquire it. There was a catch, though. Apparently, when the airplane ran out of fuel-and for that price there was no fuel gauge-it would go into a dive, and a nose first landing would be unavoidable. I was intrigued and stopped the car to take a closer look.

The product looked very much like a Second World War fighter jet and also something like a Mustang. I couldn't help being interested and made up my mind to visit the distributors showroom when we returned from our trip.

By the time we arrived back in the city it was pretty late, but the showroom was still open so we stopped by and asked for a brochure. The salesman asserted we had little time to order since their product was in great demand. I assured him I bought absolutely nothing major without first sleeping on it, and this would definitely be considered a major purchase. He finally gave me a brochure, muttering about how few they had left.

Brochure in hand, we returned to the car and made our way home. The next morning, I took some time to examine the information on

A First Step

the new low-cost aircraft. It seemed to have exciting possibilities, in spite of its tendency to be a 'one-way ticket.' The small print indicated another problem. In addition to its proclivity for landing nose first, it seems the plane screeched like a dive-bomber. The noisemaking device couldn't be switched off. To stop the racket, it had to be physically destroyed. To this end, the manufacturer had placed a small bomb in the nose of the aircraft, the cost of which was included in the selling price-thus the nickname, Flying Bombs.

The small print put me off, and I lost interest. Others, however, were obviously not deterred, for within a few weeks, the skies were full of screaming aircraft. It was hard to ignore them. All you could do was wait and hope they didn't run out of fuel while overhead.

Some time later, we were shopping downtown and saw one of the Flying Bombs. According to other shoppers, it had been aloft for a while, and everyone was anxiously eyeing the sky. Suddenly we could hear the engine cut, and the plane went into a nosedive right above the shopping area. Either deliberately or as the result of a miscalculation, the pilot had obviously run out of gas. Who will ever know?

Thankfully, he missed hitting anything but hardtop, but I became absolutely convinced that I didn't want to buy one.

...

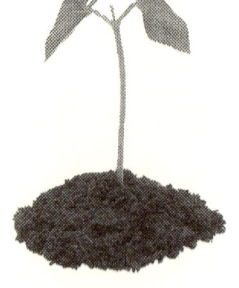

43
Across the Great Lake

I needed the treatment, so I had to travel. It was going to be very risky, yet I could not delay. My pneumonia was very much in evidence, and to get help, I had to take a boat across the Great Lake to Blueport, a small fishing town with a population of about ten thousand. I would have to arrange for someone to drive me to the harbour and help me onto the ferry. Luckily, there was no shortage of volunteers.

By the next morning, all necessary arrangements had been made, my ticket had been delivered, and Peter, one of the people I had been staying with, had offered to drive me to the dock. It must have been at least minus 5 degrees Centigrade-forty below if you considered the wind-chill factor. Peter pulled up as close to the boarding ramp as he could and, struggling through a fresh fall of snow, helped me to board. He wished me a safe journey and was on his way. In the hold, it was a little warmer, but not much.

The ferry was an unusual craft, almost circular, rather like a saucer. The accommodations were quite primitive. The passengers made a large circle, some sitting on sleeping bags, some lying down to keep warm, and others perched with their backs to a circular wall. I took the sleeping bag I'd been given, put it close to the wall, and just about collapsed onto it. It was so cold I could see my breath. Finally, the loading hatch was closed, and that helped me to feel a little warmer.

After perhaps a half an hour, we were moving. The lake was calm, and as we sailed through the harbour, there was just a gentle swell accompanied by the rhythmic hum of the engines.

There was a much larger contingent of First Nations people on board than I expected. One young lady was eyeing me with concern. She seemed to know I had a temperature, and after some time had elapsed, she came over, pulled my blanket more securely around me, and asked if there was anything she could do to help.

"You have chest pains?" she queried.

She didn't wait for me to answer. Seeing the sweat pouring from my brow, she indicated she would be straight back with a vapour rub. Within five minutes, she came back carrying a jar and a piece of cloth. She bared my chest and started to apply the jar's contents, rubbing with vigour.

"Why are you visiting our village at Thunder Mountain?" she asked. "We have no hospitals there, and you are in need of some care."

By then, I was feeling really ill. "I can get medical attention when we reach Blueport," I muttered.

"But we're not going anywhere near Blueport," she said sounding startled. We're going to Leatherhead, a small village at the foot of Thunder Mountain. You must have gotten on the wrong ferry."

That was the last thing I needed to hear. For the first time, I wondered if I were going to beat this infection. I was banking on getting treatment when the ferry docked. Now it appeared I would be ending that journey hundreds of miles from any sort of hospital or care facility.

"Don't worry," she said when she saw my reaction. "I am sure some of the elders will take you under their wing. I will talk to Chief Running Waters. He is a very compassionate man and will not want to see you in distress. He is actually travelling with us, sitting on the far side of the boat."

Hearing that relieved me some, and I summoned up a little more energy to ask the caring young lady her name. "Marina," was her reply. "I am travelling with my mother. We are returning from a shopping expedition for supplies to see us through the winter. The lake will soon be frozen over-in fact it is close to being frozen right now. If you listen, from time to time, you can hear the ice crack."

"Does that mean I am going to be stuck in Leatherhead?" My anxiety was clearly evident in my voice.

Weighing her thoughts carefully before responding, she quietly gave me encouragement. "Not really. If the Lake does freeze up-and it may not for another week or so-there would be emergency flights out to Blueport. In any case, my people will not see you alone and vulnerable." She gently wiped my forehead, and I fell asleep.

I am not sure how much later I awoke, but Marina's mother had my head cradled into her lap. I was very ill. I could sense we were nearing our destination, but had no idea how I was going to get off the ferry or where I would go. I was grateful to Marina and her mother for their attention and gained comfort from the fact that they had, apparently, taken control of my situation. I remember feeling a brief flash of concern when I heard someone say that it was so cold, it would be a miracle if I survived the crisis on this boat. Then I fell asleep again.

Suddenly, I heard chains banging against the side of the ferry and knew we must be docking. Passengers were starting to collect their belongings and tidy up their sleeping bags. No one was moving to the exits, though, and I soon learned why. Apparently, whenever it was below zero, the temperature inside the ferry had to equal that outside. It had something to do with the fact that the vessel was old. The silence following the cutting of the engines simply indicated a period of waiting for it to get colder.

Those people were right. If I get off this boat alive, it truly will be a miracle, I thought, although Marina and her mother were staying close and doing their best to nurse me and keep me warm. How lucky I was to have the attention of such good people. Without them, I guessed my chances would be close to zero.

After what seemed an eternity, the hatch was slowly opened. A freezing fog drifted around the opening as everyone started to move towards the exit. My guardian angels, as I thought of them, called on Chief Running Water for his assistance. Without hesitation, he sent over two of his sons. They were strapping young men, well built, and over six-feet tall. They laid out what appeared to be a huge bearskin, asked me to lie on it, and proceeded to lift me up and carry me off the ferry. The next thing I remembered was wak-

A First Step

ing up to find myself in a warmly furnished cabin with Marina standing over me.

"Your fever broke last night," she said. "After what you have experienced, you are very lucky to be alive. We were not sure we could save you, but some higher being had dictated that you would live. We have seen a miracle. Everybody says it's a miracle."

With some difficulty, I raised my head and enquired as to how long I had been there.

"Three days," was her reply, "but don't let that worry you. We have to get you well before you can think of doing anything else."

Reassured and feeling comfortable and warm, I watched the flicker of firelight reflecting off the exposed roof beams. I fell into another deep sleep.

The next thing I knew, someone was looking down at me. This time it was not Marina, but Sylvia. When she saw me opening my eyes and noticed I was regaining some colour in my cheeks, the sadness in her blue eyes changed to a look of relief and then happiness. She knew what that meant.

I was in my room in Intensive Care, and how I had been transported back from across the lake, I will never know. The important thing was I had beaten the pneumonia.

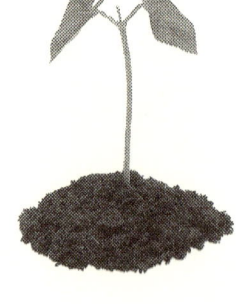

44
A Game of Chicken

Some people love to play with fire. That phrase could be literally applied to a new craze, which involved the passing around of an eighteen-inch bomb until something made it detonate. The person holding it when it exploded was obviously the loser.

On this particular day, I happened to be in the downtown mall adjoining the railroad station. The lunchtime crowd was just thinning out, and I was moving quite nimbly with no sign of Guillain-Barré Syndrome. As I made my way to the top of the escalators that divided the mall from the station, I noticed several colleagues clambering on some beams almost at the height of the roof that ran above the tracks and loading platforms. It took me a minute to see what they were up to.

Up over the heads of an unsuspecting crowd of mall staff, shoppers, railroad officials, passengers, and passers by, a serious game of chicken was being played with a bomb. Straight away I recognized two of the players as my friends Jordan and Red, so I decided to join them. It would be a bit of harmless fun, or so I thought at the time.

Red had the bomb. The way he was handling it told me it was live. He was hanging by his legs from a roof beam holding the bomb by its fins. The object of the rather dangerous game was to keep passing the bomb around without ever letting it touch the ground. If you were left holding the bomb at the end of the day, or worse, if you accidentally dropped it, you were in big trouble.

Red had slowly inched over to where Jordan and several of his friends were waiting. At one point he would be climbing; at another point, he would be traversing roof beams until he got close enough to another player to attempt a pass off. I made the decision to take the next pass, figuring that since there were quite a few participants and it was early afternoon, it was unlikely I would be left with no one to pass to.

Quickly scaling the framework of the station concourse, I reached Red; but I was just a little late, and he had already passed the bomb. Clambering over girders high above the station, I tried to anticipate the intended destination of the guy who now had it so that I could intercept him and take a pass. It took longer than I would have liked, but eventually I caught up with him.

I decided to take the game to a lower level. Holding the bomb in one hand and being careful to avoid letting it touch any surface, I reached the side framework and slowly descended from the roof level to the shopping mall ceiling. At just that moment, a train came rumbling through the station.

Three heavy diesel locomotives were pulling perhaps a hundred cars fully loaded with freight. The vibrations made it essential to hang on tightly, all the time keeping the bomb from touching either the side framework or me. That was easier said than done, and I was soon covered in perspiration.

Red, Jordan and others were watching me intently and were obviously pleased to be simply onlookers with such a major distraction as the freight train passing through. I couldn't let go of my handhold, so I just had to wait for the freight, which was most definitely taking its time. Finally, after what seemed like an eternity, the last car passed, and with it, the noise and distraction. Now, I had to decide my next move.

My hold on the ledge was getting insecure. I decided to move across towards Jordan. He had been moving gradually in my direction, and I hoped his intention was to take a pass. I could then take a badly needed breather.

Sure enough, Jordan accepted the bomb, and grinned from ear to ear as he said approvingly, "You have guts!"

...

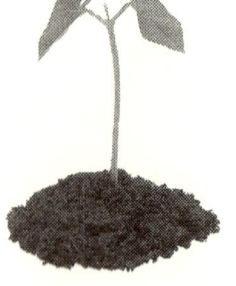

45
Jet Fighters On Call

* * *

It was a beautiful warm day in early fall. There were eight or nine jet fighters parked, nose first, in the trees opposite my room. Backed by tall conifers, some of the trees had been planted when the grounds of the hospital were initially landscaped a good number of years ago. Mostly they were green-leafed varieties, including some heavily berried Mountain Ash; but there were also quite a number of a red-leafed variety, and it was these that the jet pilots seemed to prefer to use as their stand-by locations.

The pilots, in goggles and full flying gear, were either sitting in their aircraft or standing on a branch alongside. In any event, they were ready for action. How they backed out and made their way to a runway when the call came, I never knew. I did see how they landed, though. They'd come straight into a tree and stop, perfectly balanced, among the branches!

I had heard there was a new airport a few blocks away and wondered if this were some kind of publicity stunt. Since Sylvia and I would be departing from the new airport on a trip to Spain, we would possibly soon find out.

Time passed, and it was another sunny day, quite hot for the time of year. We made our way to the airport. We were walking, and it was uphill most of the way, which must have been tough for Sylvia, since she was pushing me in my wheelchair. We hadn't booked a flight, since it was cheaper to take advantage of the airline's introductory

A First Step

plan, which involved simply entering your names at check-in for the next flight to your destination. There was a snag, though.

This introductory offer applied only to six-seater twin-engine aircraft; so, allowing for a pilot, that left room for five passengers. If more than five people were listed for a flight, a drawing would be held to determine who could board.

When Sylvia and I arrived at the check-in desk, we were directed to wait in the lounge. Imagine our surprise when we spotted two of our friends there, also waiting for a flight to Spain. We enjoyed the great view and basked in the sunshine that was streaming in through the large windows. I was so comfortable that I fell asleep.

The next thing I remember was being gently awakened. The sun was still shining, but something was different. When I looked out the window, the trees with the red leaves and the Mountain Ash loaded with their red berries were still there, but no airport. The jet fighters that had been parked in the trees had also disappeared, and I was no longer in a wheelchair, but back in the hospital again. I don't know what happened to our trip to Spain!

...

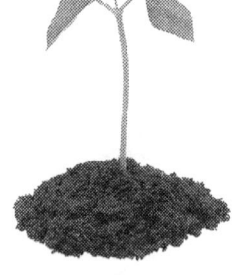

46
Wild Dogs Attack

We were making good progress on our drive home from Ottawa. The weather was ideal for travelling, and we were getting close to Swift Current, Saskatchewan. While driving over the prairie, both Sylvia and I had observed small off-white animals. Sometimes they were in pairs; then at other times, they'd be in larger packs. On one occasion there must have been at least a dozen of them chasing a coyote. They looked a little like dogs-and perhaps they were wild dogs, but we had only seen them at a distance, so it was difficult to tell.

Now, with the prairie and its animals behind us, we were concentrating on finding a place to gas up and have a snack. I was ready for a drink. Driving always made me thirsty, rather than hungry.

We soon came upon signs welcoming visitors to Swift Current, population 14,000, and within minutes, came upon familiar signs advertising filling stations. Selecting one which had a restaurant alongside, I pulled into the forecourt, gassed up, parked the car, and Sylvia and I went in search of some food. When we entered the restaurant, it became immediately evident that there were many intense discussions going on. As we were led to one of the few vacant tables, our waitress turned to us exclaiming, "It's awful, isn't it?"

"What is?" I asked.

"Haven't you heard about the wild dogs roaming around in huge packs and attacking people?" She pointed towards a window table. "The couple sitting over there saw them get two teenage boys riding their bikes near Gull Lake. They actually dragged the boys off the bikes and killed them. Other people have also seen some awful things. It's getting really scary."

A First Step

I mentioned we had come in from Manitoba and had seen a few dogs, but nothing like the large packs she was describing."

"I'm not surprised," she replied. "These dogs seem to be coming into Saskatchewan from Alberta, where, apparently, they have been a real plague. I hear they are out of control, particularly in Central Alberta."

"That is real bad news," I told her, explaining that we were on our way to Calgary and would have to go through that area. She sympathised as she took our order.

We talked it over and decided that, come what may, we would just have to keep going. Our snack arrived and with it the additional piece of advice to be extra cautious going through the Maple Creek area. Apparently, that is where the largest packs had been sighted. Neither Sylvia nor I said much as we ate. It was enough that everyone else appeared to be chattering nervously. From the overheard conversation, we were not the only ones to be headed west.

I paid the bill, and we returned to the car. Everyone we passed wished us good luck. It sounded as though we would need it.

Back on the highway, the very next area we would be passing through was Gull Lake, where the wild dogs had attacked the cyclists. Several times we thought we saw packs of them in the distance. Then suddenly, there they were! They were still some distance ahead, but they were definitely in our path. It was a huge pack, numbering perhaps forty or fifty dogs. The animals were just milling around on the highway. We covered the distance with our hearts in our mouth, but fortunately, right before we reached the pack, their attention was drawn away from the highway by two farm dogs, one a German shepherd and the other something like a Pit Bull.

We had to look the other way as we passed by. The farm dogs didn't stand a chance. The wild dogs only stood ten to twelve inches high, but they had a wide bulldog type stance and lethal looking teeth and jaws, which they did not hesitate to use.

Once we got beyond those repulsive, marauding animals, the prairie scene seemed almost pastoral, and we tried to forget what we had seen. The road ahead appeared to be clear, but for how long we could only guess. Mile after mile passed, and for the better part of half an hour, there was only the odd sighting of small groups of the off-white coloured dogs, and thankfully, none were on the road. I wondered how I would react if a pack did indeed block the highway and refuse to move. I would not turn around, so other than stopping and waiting them out, the only option would be to plough through them. That could get ugly, and I didn't want to think about it.

Gull Lake was now behind us, and we were fast approaching Maple Creek, the area we had been warned about. Everything seemed normal, however. The sky was blue and we could see clear to the horizon. It was a beautiful day and we were making good time. Surely nothing could go wrong. *I must have had a bad dream*, I thought. How else could I explain the nightmarish threat posed by the wild dogs?

Then I knew this was no dream. I saw something I will never forget. In the distance, the horizon was actually throbbing! Instinctively, I knew the movement was created by hordes of the off-white dogs. Sylvia had fallen into a comfortable sleep, no doubt lulled by the purring of the engine and the warmth of the day. That was good. *Maybe with luck we will get through the next part of the journey without her having to be alarmed*, I thought. Bracing myself, I drove on.

For the next fifty or so kilometres the road was clear. The marauding animals were very much in evidence, though, and it seemed only a matter of time before they would confront us. When we reached the western edge of Maple Creek, we encountered what we had dreaded. There were dogs all over the road—perhaps hundreds of them- and these were in no better humour than the ones we had seen earlier.

A pack of a dozen or more had encircled a couple walking their pet Scottie. We made it past, but what I saw in the rear-view mirror turned my stomach. More of the horrible off-white creatures had arrived on the scene, and as though pre-planned and co-ordinated, the whole mass launched a ferocious attack on the terrified puppy. Its owners were not spared either, and there was absolutely nothing anyone could do to help them.

I moved gingerly forward, and thankfully the dogs moved aside as I proceeded through the intersection. I saw their giving ground more as self preservation than backing down and was grateful for my large, solid car. On the other side of the intersection, a guy in a white convertible was fighting a losing battle against the dozens of dogs that were jumping into his car and viciously attacking him. Again, there was nothing I could do but keep going.

Slowly picking up speed, I continued working my way through the packs of animals. I took comfort in the fact that, by now, a number of other vehicles were also travelling west behind me. I was glad not to be alone and, fortunately, Sylvia had slept through the whole episode.

After leaving Maple Creek, there were fewer of the wild dogs, but we still had to be very vigilant. By the time we reached the Calgary city limits, I had struck and possibly killed three or four. In view of their sheer numbers, it was surprising I hadn't hit more of them.

I decided to stop in at the office, which was on the way home. By this time, we were again surrounded by numerous packs of the wild animals. They were on both sides of the highway, and when we turned off to approach the office parking lot, there were more of them on both sides of the road. In fact, there were dogs as far as the eye could see. The only exception was that there were no dogs in the parking lot itself, although there were a few across the road, and they seemed quite interested in our arrival.

Sylvia did not want to stay in the car by herself, so we decided we should both make a run across the ten or so yards between our car and the office door. I inched in a little closer, cutting the distance by about three yards. We agreed to exit the car on a count of three, then opened our doors simultaneously and made a dash for safety. We were just in time. As I got through behind Sylvia, the two lead dogs were throwing themselves against the now closing doors. That was too close for comfort.

Inside, there was pandemonium. Some of the wild dogs had broken in through a back door. They were, for the moment, contained, but we could hear them clawing and scratching and throwing themselves against walls and doors in search of a weak spot where they could break through.

Then we discovered they had a weak spot! On their forehead, cen-

Wild Dogs Attack

trally positioned above eye level, there was a protuberance. Several people had noted that if a dog was threatened with a stake or iron bar to the head, the animal would freeze, open it's eyes wide, and appear to say 'oh no, please don't'. One fellow was seen to take pity on a dog and back off. He did not have long to regret his decision. As soon as lowered his weapon, the animal leaped on him and sank its fangs into his throat.

If the dogs took a blow to the protuberance, however, they were instantly felled; so, everyone in the building had armed himself with a stake or club of some sort.

Sylvia and I spent several hours helping the others beat off any dogs that broke through. After a while, things quietened down somewhat, and I decided we had better head for home. There was no telling what we would find there.

Choosing our moment carefully, Sylvia and I made a dash for our car and lost no time getting underway. It struck us as strange, but the farther south we travelled, the fewer wild dogs we encountered.

It took us about thirty minutes to get home. There were no wild dogs in sight. In fact, we had seen none for the last two or three kilometres. Very much relieved, Sylvia went indoors and I started to unpack the car. After what we had just experienced, the calm seemed very quiet and unreal. I had taken one load in and was in the midst of bringing in another when I heard a shout. I looked up just in time to see two of the ferocious dogs bearing down on me.

I darted towards the open front door and almost made it. Then, to my horror, I felt a searing pain in my right leg. That was the first indication that one of the dogs had drawn blood. I managed to reached the house and pulled the door closed behind me with not a second to spare. Safely inside, I limped into the kitchen to examine my injured leg. Sylvia took one look and insisted I got to the Emergency Room for treatment. After a brief moment's thought, I agreed and phoned for an ambulance.

Half an hour later, I was at Rockyview Hospital. I saw many of the nurses I knew from the Intensive Care Unit and figured they must have been called in because of the wild dog crisis. If I had imagined that, because I was an existing patient, they would come to my aid quickly, I was mistaken. Much to my annoyance, I had to wait my turn. I flagged down one of the nurses and tried to get some idea of how much longer I would have to be patient.

"Brian," she said sharply, "we have so many people here who are in much worse shape than you. We will be with you as soon as we can." I felt a little abashed at the upbraiding, but guess I deserved it.

I don't recall how long I had to wait, but finally, Stephanie came over and playfully scolded me for my impatience. She wheeled me over to another room where, with help, I was transferred to a bed. Once my wounds were cleaned and dressed, Stephanie called for a porter to take me back to Intensive Care. She must have wondered how I had managed to get my leg torn up by a wild dog without leaving the hospital, but she never asked.

...

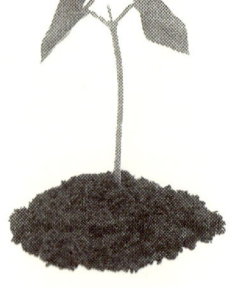

47
Catastrophe

It was one of those ordinary Sundays. Sylvia and I had decided to take a short drive and find somewhere different to enjoy a leisurely cup of coffee. The weather, though, was anything but ordinary. The day had started sunny and warm, but then turned thundery. Next a weather system came through, bringing high winds followed by lots of rain. Before long, the temperature dropped, and the rain changed to sleet. Finally, it started to snow.

As we set off, the sun was peeking through the clouds, but with all the moisture in the air, it was becoming quite misty. In fact, before we had traveled very far, the weather forecasters would probably be calling it 'fog.' We decided not to venture too far, and headed for the Midnapore Railway Station, where there was a reasonably good restaurant on the upper level.

Arriving at the station, which actually no longer served as one since passenger trains didn't come through anymore, I parked the car. By this time visibility was perhaps only a hundred yards or so. We made our way inside, hoping that by the time we came out, things would have improved.

In the station, very little was left on the ground floor except an empty ticket office and waiting room. We were just about to head up the flight of concrete steps that led to the second floor restaurant, when I had a strange sense of foreboding. Maybe this was not a good idea. I was about to suggest we choose another restaurant when my attention was drawn to a lady who appeared somewhat distressed. Sylvia noticed her too. We went to offer assistance.

"How can we help?" Sylvia asked as we approached her.

A First Step

"My car has broken down," she told us in broken English. "I am a visitor to this country and thought I would be able to continue my journey by train."

"No passenger trains travel this line," I explained. "This building hasn't functioned as a station in years. It serves a different purpose now."

"No one told me that," she sighed. "I have been waiting since early this morning."

This made our next decision easy. "Please allow us to buy you some food and a warm drink," I offered. Afterwards I will drive you to the Greyhound Bus Terminal."

The lady gratefully accepted the offer and asked us to wait while she went back to her car for something. No sooner had she left us than we heard the unmistakable sound of powerful diesel engines rumbling towards us through the fog. Soon we could make out a headlight, and the ground was starting to vibrate. I could not help but be in awe of the huge locomotives that were capable of hauling so much freight, particularly when lashed together in threes and fours, as trains on this line so often were.

I hoped the lady, whose name we still had not discovered, would have the good sense to stay on her side of the track until the train passed by. It couldn't be far away now, but the fog made it difficult to judge just how close it was. Soon the noise was pounding at the eardrums, and the ground was trembling under the weight and momentum of the heavy diesels. The train was now emerging from the fog and approaching the station fairly rapidly, no doubt picking up speed as it was leaving the city.

Both Sylvia and I stood watching as the first of the locomotives thundered through. It was an impressive sight. Then came the repetitive sounds of the freight cars passing by. I had, on many previous occasions, counted one hundred or more in a single train, and this one seemed to be no exception. We decided to head up the stairs to the restaurant, thinking we would find a table, then, after the freight had passed, I could come down to find the lady we had offered to help.

On entering the restaurant, there was a tremendous noise, and the whole building shook violently. I ran down the stairs to see

··· *Catastrophe* ···

what was happening and, to my amazement, saw that one of the freight cars had a wide load that had not only hit the side of the building, but had lifted it off its foundation and was dragging it along, carrying us down the track like a projectile. I considered making a jump to safety, but couldn't do that without Sylvia, so I let the opportunity pass. We were now traveling at a high speed, as if caught in a huge spinning top, yet the inside where we were, was absolutely stationary.

I rushed back upstairs, where there was something of a pandemonium. Everyone was looking out the windows in utter disbelief. Here we were in an urban restaurant, yet the rest of the world was rushing by at an alarming speed. The rail line from Midnapore going south was on a downhill gradient. The engineer, who I doubted had any knowledge of the extra baggage he'd picked up, was increasing power, and we were now traveling like a bullet.

For about twenty kilometres we moved in a line that was more or less straight. Then the track curved westward. It was at this point that the train and the station parted company. When the locomotive banked into the curve, the station continued in the direction it had been going, and was now sailing along on its own without any loss of speed.

We had no idea where this was all going to end. Prospects became darker when the restaurant manager turned on the radio just in time to hear a news bulletin on the 'Midnapore Disaster'.

"Hope is not yet lost for those trapped inside the station," the voice on the radio announced, "though the building is now traveling south-south east, leaving a trail of destruction in its wake. Officials say chances of a successful rescue operation are becoming increasingly remote, but experts are doing their best to come up with a plan."

That was how the general populace was learning of our predicament. They were told the likelihood was that we would finish up in a small lake or river and be unable to exit the building. The anchorman explained that the best-case scenario was that the building would end up in the marshes where the water wasn't deep enough to cause drowning, but that the occupants might starve before rescuers could reach them. Although the outlook seemed pretty grim, we were trying to remain upbeat.

There were ten other people, including the restaurant's day manager, on board this fast moving projectile. Interestingly, almost everyone had a story about how they almost didn't choose this restaurant on this particular day. Only one elderly couple appeared resigned to their fate. To relieve the tension, the manager announced that all food and drink were now on the house. It did help a little. Then someone spotted a rescue helicopter flying overhead. That was good to see, although we realized not much could be done until we came to rest somewhere.

On and on we went, though we were losing some speed. I looked out the window in time to see us smash through the gate at a railway crossing and then careen down a well-traveled roadway. Thankfully we avoided hitting any cars. I decided to check out the damage downstairs, and scope things out just in case we needed a quick exit once this thing stopped. The manager agreed we should be prepared and offered to come with me.

We went through the swinging doors and cautiously made our way down the first flight of stairs. Everything looked normal until we got to the landing midway down. There we were confronted by chaos. Where the outer doors used to be there was nothing but soil, vegetation, tree branches, rocks, and other debris that had been collected on our devastating run. There was no sign of the doors themselves, nor could we see any possible escape route. The exit was totally plugged.

"I've seen enough," I told the manager. "Let's see how we end up when we stop. If we come to a violent halt, perhaps enough damage will be done to give us an escape route."

He agreed, obviously hoping, as I was, that escape would be possible in the end. "What shall we tell the others?" he asked me.

"Lets tell them the truth-that it's a mess down here and we won't know much until we see how we finish up. Who knows? In the end, there may be several escape routes open to us."

The bizarre trip seemed endless. Now we were obviously on the prairie, since everywhere we looked, the land was flat and feature-

Catastrophe

less. Our speed was still decreasing, but slowly; and the end of our run was nowhere in sight. We had no idea what was powering our movement now that we were free of the freight train.

The radio program was again interrupted to update listeners on our plight. It was eerie to be hearing the details of a catastrophe of which we were a part. Our path was apparently being tracked via reports phoned in by the ranchers and farmers whose properties we were crossing. Speculation was rife that the station would end up in the Drumhead Marshes, which would make rescue extremely difficult, if not impossible. We tried not to dwell on such a gloomy thought. "Anything could happen," we told ourselves.

Suddenly the scenery changed. We appeared to be headed into a large gully, and the level tabletop of the prairie was now above us. The deeper we went, the wider apart were the defining walls. It was beginning to appear that the gully was turning into a much larger canyon. The references on the radio to our finishing up in the marshes or in a lake now seemed to make sense.

As we headed downward into the canyon we must have gained some momentum, but we were now starting to level out again. Hopefully that meant we would be slowing down. I noticed the ground cover was becoming lush, which indicated the presence of moisture. I wondered if this were the marshy country that had been referred to in the radio alerts. It seemed we were about to find out.

The ride was becoming decidedly smoother at this point. Then, without any warning, everyone was thrown violently across the restaurant. Finally, we had stopped. A quick check turned up no major injuries, though most of us were hurting.

Now we had to find an escape route. I went to the doors and found them jammed, but when several of us charged with our shoulders, one of them swung aside. I ran through and headed down the stairs. As I had hoped, we'd gone into a rocky outcrop and the force of the collision had split one of the outside walls. There appeared to be enough space to crawl through. *But what about the ground outside*, I wondered? I decided to check it out, which proved to be a good decision. After making my way to the gap and peering out, all I could see was water. It was difficult to judge how deep it was and that presented a definite problem, but I calculated that we could not be far from the rocks and dry land.

I turned to the manager, who had come to look for himself.

"There must be a broom in the cleaning cupboard," I suggested. "We could use it to check the depth of the water." He agreed and offered to get it.

We soon determined that the water was about three feet deep. Now it might be possible to make plans. By this time, everyone had come to view the potential escape route, but it was soon agreed we should wait and see if rescuers came. Our wild ride had obviously been monitored so our whereabouts would soon be known, if we hadn't already been spotted.

Then someone shouted, "Look! Water is coming in."

Sure enough, water was now pouring in through the split in the wall. This was a new and worrisome development. Everyone must have been thinking, as I was: *How deep are we going to settle? Could it block our escape route?* It was then that one of the girls on the restaurant level spotted our would-be rescuers through the window.

We would still have to wait a while, but a party of six or seven was, indeed, scaling down an escarpment towards us. They were carrying planks and an assortment of ropes so their progress was rather slow. In the meantime, I tried to get a fix on where we were from the radio, but unfortunately, when we crashed it had fallen to the floor and no longer worked.

It took some time for us all to evacuate the station, but eventually, with the assistance of our rescuers and their equipment, we waded through three feet of water to relatively dry land. We made our way along the base of the cliff, which led us to a fault in the side of the canyon, and from there, through a cutting where we were able to climb to the upper level.

Upon reaching the prairie, we saw that situated in a depression about half a mile away was a hotel that had an excellent view of the canyon. That was a pleasant surprise, or so it appeared at the time. *We can surely get help there*, I thought. I mentioned it to our rescuers and they agreed. We needed dry clothes and, more importantly, needed to shower. Wading waist deep in muddy water had left its mark on all of us. *Surely in view of our predicament, the hotel management would not refuse to help.*

The closer we got, however, the more obvious it became that we were looking at a luxury resort. That raised the question as to whether an upscale establishment would want to accommodate such a rag tag group as we. We would soon find out. There was very little alternative, so we had to press on and take our chances. By this time our clothes had thoroughly dried, but the evidence of our wading through the marsh could not be so easily hidden.

We reached the hotel entrance and decided to bite the bullet and enter the lobby. I saw the look on the face of one of the receptionists as we approached. It was not encouraging. She immediately came out from behind the front desk and hustled us into a side office. When we explained what had happened she looked like she didn't believe us. "We are fully booked for the season," she said with a somewhat icy tone. "The only rooms in which we could accommodate you are the staff quarters in the basement."

It was getting late, and we were all tired. "That's good enough for me," I responded. "As long as there is a bed to sleep on, I will gladly take one of the staff rooms." Everyone else echoed my sentiments, and after the receptionist cleared the arrangements with her manager, we were led downstairs to our respective rooms.

It did not take long to fall asleep that night.

Suddenly, I could feel someone gently shaking my shoulder. I opened my eyes, looked up, and saw a nurse. "Wake up, it's time for your blanket bath." Just for a moment, I wondered where I was. Then I realized I was back in my hospital room. I did not remember who had brought me back or how. Another thing puzzled me. How was it that no one appeared to miss me or, if they did, once again chose to say nothing about it? Don't they check the beds for patients every night?

* * *

Photos for Chapter 27, "GBS Patient on a Secret Mission"

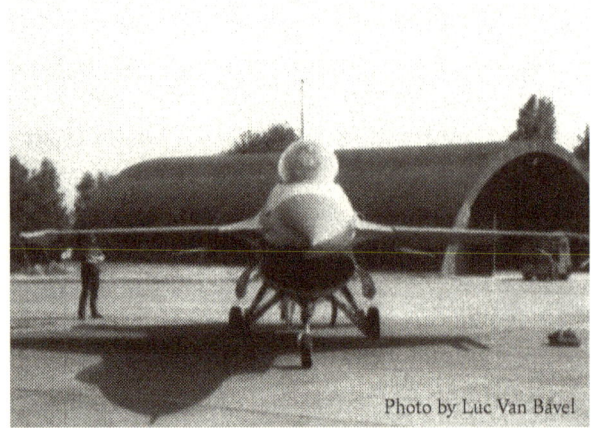

The F-16 of my dreams.

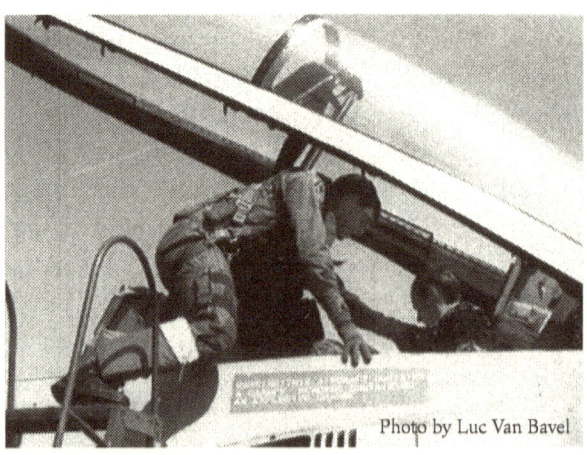

This could be the Wing Commander going over the controls with me, but in fact it was "Sprengy" and Luc of the Belgium Air Force.

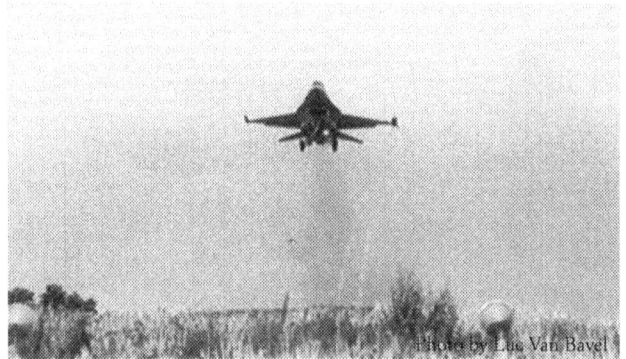

Take-off!

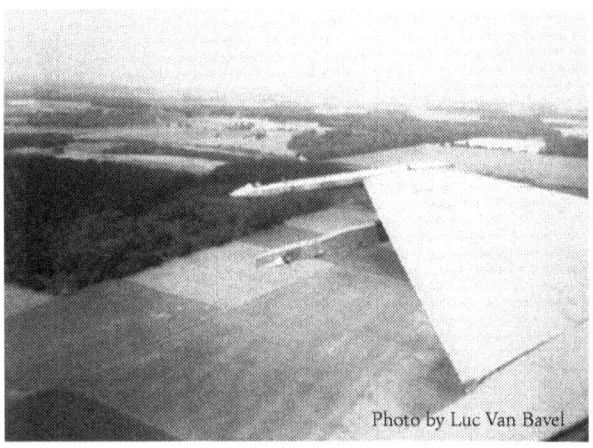

After successfully flying around for about half an hour, I decide to bring the aircraft back to base.

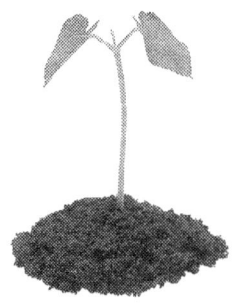

Part III
Epilogue

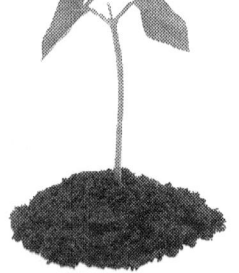

Epilogue
Leaving the Dream World Behind

❊ ❊ ❊

I've left the dream world behind. Three and a half years after succumbing to GBS, life is gradually returning to something close to normal. Except for a weakness in my hands and feet, my health is generally very good — some may say excellent — and I continue to experience improvement, although at a very slow rate. This means I can expect the daily tasks like getting dressed, which so many of us take for granted, to become easier as time goes on. I can do a little to help my caregivers, but not everything. I can manage a spoon and fork, but a knife? Not yet.

I still need a wheelchair a lot of the time, but am lucky to have an extremely manoeuvrable electric-powered model. It is a comfortable computer 'task chair' for one thing! It also fits quite snugly under our kitchen table at mealtimes. Otherwise, I am moving around either with a walker or independently — when I can find the arm of a willing volunteer. My next goal is to use a cane. The longer-term goals I spoke of in Part 1 have not changed; they are just taking a little longer to achieve.

Goals are important. Without them, new accomplishments may never be achieved. It is all too easy to accept things as they are and just get by. As physiotherapists have told me many times, "If you don't use it, you'll lose it!"

To achieve the goals that I keep setting for myself, I continue to follow a fairly strict exercise program, both at home and at the University of Calgary, currently aided and abetted by Carol — the first caregiver to succeed in putting on and lacing up a left shoe on my right foot before I noticed — and by Helen, my physiotherapist.

On a spiritual note, I have to wonder if the things that happen in our lives happen for a purpose. Since becoming sick, I have crossed paths with some wonderful people — people my wife and I would probably never have met had our life continued on its former path.

Then there are all those wonderful family members, friends, and acquaintances who continually assist and support us in ways we never expected. My wife's hairdresser, for example, has offered to come to our home to cut my hair whenever necessary. Our neighbours shovel the driveway after each snow and, in the summer, cut the lawn when a cut is needed. Valued and true friends include Sylvia in their outings, giving her a much-needed 'time out.' The 'pros' at Priddis made up a weighted, shortened golf club so I could practise my swing.

One hears so much bad news these days. I, on the other hand, have been overwhelmed by good news and by the goodness and generosity of people of all ages, professions, and creeds.

I hope this book will be an inspiration to all who come into contact with Guillain-Barré Syndrome, whether as a patient, a relative or a caregiver.

··· The Author···

...

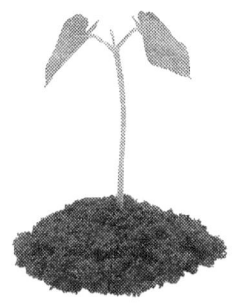

Part IV
Appendices
Endnotes, Support & Information
Resources, Reading List,
Biography, and Index

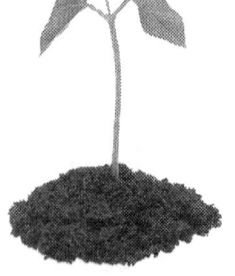

Appendix 1
Endnotes

1. Steinberg, *GBS — An Overview for the Lay Person*, published by the Guillain-Barré Syndrome Foundation International, 1998, p. 3

2. Ibid.

3. Ibid.

4. Winer, *The Early Years, Reaching Out*, Published by the GBS Support Group of the UK, April 1995, p.5

5. Ibid.

6. Ibid.

7. Steinberg, pp. 3,4.

8. Ibid, pp. 4,5.

9. Ibid.

10. Ibid, pp 5,6,7

11. Ibid, pp 6,7.

12. Burk, *New Jersey Medicine*, Jan 1989, Vol. 86, No. 1, pp. 50-51.

13. I recall being afraid of being left on my own. Barely able to move and communicate with anyone, if, for example, I were to experience extreme discomfort, breathing difficulties, or become disconnected from the ventilator, I could not summon assistance, or so I imagined, ignoring the fact that I was closely monitored. (Author).

14. This was a 'Peripherally Inserted Central Catheter' (Author)

15. Burk, *New Jersey Medicine*, 1989, Vol. 86, No. 1, Pp 50-51

16. Soccer team in the English Premier Division supported by my brother and I since we were kids.

17. Being unable to use my hands, the blue hat, which was a baseball cap, with a pointer affixed to the peak, provided a way for me to point to 'word cards'. I was not very keen on the idea, as it tended to be error-prone. I think I may have 'lost' it!

18. *Evening Post*, Nov 10, 1998, P11.

19. I found the ventilator alarm to be quite a pleasant sound. So much so, that on hearing it again while on a social visit to the Rockyview ICU over 18 months later, it brought back memories of a time when I was being cared for and visited by some wonderful people.

20. A trach cork is a plastic plug which is used to

Appendix 1: Endnotes

plug the tracheal tube, after the trach insert — an inner cannula — is replaced with a 'fenestrated' insert which has a hole in it for airflow, allowing the patient to breath room air normally through the nose and throat, and allow phonation, whilst free of the ventilator. (Author)

21. A trach cradle is a cradle, or mask, that covers the trach opening, allowing moisture (humidity) to be added to air breathed in directly through the trach opening, compensating for the moisture added to air within the nasal passages and throat in normal breathing. (Author)

22. When given the opportunity to speak, I instinctively took the chair's roll as though at a board meeting, thanked everyone for all they were doing, and kept an upbeat theme going throughout the remainder of the meeting, giving no one a chance to give me, or anyone else, any unpleasant news. For this reason, I suspect future family conferences were formatted differently.

23. Due to being in isolation, a real Christmas tree was out of the question, so Ruth, with help from the grandchildren, pasted a floor to ceiling green coloured cutout of a spruce tree on the wall, adding many homemade decorations to complete the picture. It 'wowed' me, the staff, and visitors alike.

24. I was on oxygen some of the time when not on the ventilator. The need for oxygen, although in reduced quantities, continued through to the early physiotherapy sessions in the rehabilitation program at Foothills Hospital.

... *A First Step* ...

25. Chinook is the name given to winds often experienced in Southern Alberta, which carry warmer Pacific air from the west, surfacing after crossing the Rocky Mountains.

26. An urban park within the Calgary city limits, possibly the largest in Canada.

27. As I recall, the respiratory therapists, in cahoots with the nursing staff, had drawn up a graph to record my progress breathing on my own. The desired target for this day was six hours. The doctor came into my room, looked at the chart, turned to me and issued a challenge to double the day's target. I accepted and proceeded to beat it.

28. A cot is a mechanical transfer device, consisting of a canvas sheet, which is then attached by cables to the arm of the transfer stand. The patient is rolled onto it and lifted, much like a sack of potatoes, and transferred to a chair. If, as in my case, the patient is partly paralysed, the drawing together of the cables on lifting scrunches the unfortunate individual, causing legs and feet to be bent, knees forced up to chin, and the coming together of other parts of the body that were never intended to meet! (Author)

29. Finally off the ventilator after seven long months! When I was told in the morning that they were short of a ventilator and would have to take mine, I was somewhat apprehensive until they assured me that if my need became urgent, equipment would somehow be found. Much later, I learned the doctors and nurses had conspired to create a

Appendix 1: Endnotes

need for my ventilator to help me make the break! (Author)

30. It was to be June when finally discharged for good. (Author)

31. Hardly surprising, in view of the rarity of the Syndrome and the differing symptoms and recovery characteristics exhibited by G.B.S. patients. (Author)

32. G.B.S. is supposedly a rare disease, which probably explains why a few on the nursing staff appeared not to be aware of the differences between G.B.S. patients and quadriplegics or paraplegics. (Author)

33. After my test, the doctor admitted that she was not expecting a good outcome and was preparing herself to let me down gently. "Instead," she said, "you give me this great result. It is wonderful." (Author)

34. Winer, p. 5.

35. Ibid.

36. Ibid.

37. Sixteen months later, I was still trying to keep my balance standing upright without support. I am finally making some progress. This causes me to wonder if more attention should have been paid to the question of balance in the months following those first attempts. (The Author)

38. Handi-bus is the name for Calgary's transportation

system for the handicapped. I gather it is one of the best of its type in North America, both in respect of cost and efficiency. Most of the drivers excel in providing a compassionate and reliable service. Patients at the Foothills Hospital often made fun at the scheduling glitches and were impatient when buses were late; but when one considered the service makes hundreds of trips and experiences a large number of cancellations on a daily basis, they do as good a job as can be expected.

39. We were lucky to have Giselle as my first daytime caregiver. She was intelligent, caring, and had a wonderful sense of humour. I knew we would click when, on returning with me from one of the first outpatient sessions at the hospital, she mischievously wrote her name in the dust that had collected on the window of my car. That really clinched it.

40. There was no doubt in my mind that government cuts in health-care funding were responsible for cutbacks affecting both the number of staff available and equipment at their disposal. (Author)

41. Was this a dream, or was it closer to reality? I later learned from my family, that beds in the ICU at the Foothills Hospital could be enclosed by drapes, for privacy.

42. Even after nine or ten months of hospitalization, I could, on occasion, feel that my knees were bent and my lower legs were dangling with my feet almost on the floor. It was impossible of course; yet I could still see my toes at the end of the bed! I never told anyone.

... Appendix 1: Endnotes ...

43. I realize in my condition I may have been unknowingly receiving attention.

44. Dwayne is one of my sons-in-law (Author)

45. See 'Wild Dogs Attack' (Author)

46. Respiratory Therapist's Service Vehicle, which only existed in my dreams. (Author)

47. A system of above street level covered walkways and bridges connecting much of the downtown core.

48. I was to hear this a lot. It was not until visiting Rockyview ICU socially about two years later that I made the connection. The musical car horn was in fact the ventilator alarm sounding in the ward.

49. See Dream Sequence "GBS Patient on Secret Mission".

50. I discovered in later conversations with family members that there had actually been such a notice displayed in my room.

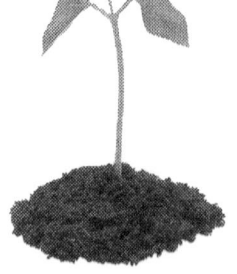

Appendix 2
Support Resources

The following are associations, organizations, and support groups that offer GBS support, information, and resources to sufferers and families contending with GBS. This is not a comprehensive listing but it is a list of the foremost. From these international resources, one is able to find further resources pertaining to their particular situations or locale. The best utilization of the resources is online at their websites. Many of these resources contain hundreds of links.

Thanks to each of the facilitators, web administrators, and contributors for the use of this information. It is because of you that people with GBS and their families are able to connect globally to conquer this terrible condition. The following information is taken directly from the listed websites and has not been altered except in presentation. Every attempt has been made to ensure the credibility and accuracy of the following information.

Guillain-Barré Syndrome Foundation International
   P.O. Box 262, Wynnewood, PA 19096
   Voice: 610-667-0131
   Fax: 610-667-7036
   Email: gbint@ix.netcom.com
   Website: http://www.guillain-barre.com/

   About the Foundation
   - The organization was founded in 1981 by Robert & Estelle Benson to help others deal with this

frightening and potentially catastrophic disorder from which recovery is uncertain. The Foundation has over 150 chapters in the United States, Canada, Europe, Australia and South Africa. Its goals are to help you, the GBS patient and family. The Foundation is proud to have on its Medical Advisory Board some of the world's leading experts on GBS as well as physicians who themselves have had the disorder.

- If you have GBS or know someone who does and would like assistance or information, contact the Foundation. If you would like to form a local support group chapter, or if you are a health care professional and would like literature or emotional support for your patients, feel free to contact us. We are here to serve you.

Services Available
- Visits to patients by recovered persons

- Comprehensive booklet, "GBS, An Overview for the Layperson"

- Handbook for Caregivers

- Discussion Boards

- Patient assistance by local chapters

- List of chapters worldwide

- Newsletter: *The Communicator*

- Research Funding

··· *Appendix 2: Support Resources* ···

- International Educational Symposia for the medical community and general public

Additional Info
- *Handbook For Caregivers*
  We are pleased to be able to present the latest in our efforts in addressing the needs of the GBS patient. A "Handbook For Caregivers", written by the wife of a GBS'er, is now available. If you would like us to mail you a copy, please complete our Request Form Online or call 610-667-0131.

- *GBS Discussion Online Forums*
  Create your own opportunity to share and compare your Guillain-Barré experience by becoming part of our on-line chapter of the Foundation. Over 150 international chapters contribute to the boards, providing an excellent opportunity to visit, share experiences, offer and receive assistance and communicate with other patients and their families.

Guillain-Barré Syndrome Support Group UK/RoI
Registered UK Charity No 327314
GBS Support Group, LCC Offices,
Eastgate, Sleaford, NG34 7EB
Tel/Fax: 01529 304615 (UK)
Int'l: (+44)1529 304615
Support helpline: 0800 374 803 (UK)
0044 1529 415278 (RoI)
E-mail: admin@gbs.org.uk
Website: http://www.gbs.org.uk/

About the Support Group

We provide information and support to all those suffering from the Guillain-Barré syndrome (GBS) and related conditions (including CIDP), and to their families and friends.

Our support activities encompass both the United Kingdom and the Republic of Ireland. Visitors to this site from other countries are most welcome to read and download our information and make use of the site's other facilities such as our on-line Forum and Guestbook.

Anyone is welcome to join the Group, but if you are seeking support and live outside the UK or RoI, we strongly suggest that in the first instance you contact a support group in your own country should one exist. Please go to our Links' page to find details of international groups.

We provide information about the GBS family of neuropathies to health professionals in the UK and the RoI. We also will give awareness presentations to groups of health professionals/students in the UK and RoI on request.

List of Services

- Extensive Website

- Annual Conference

- Conference Reports

- Telephone Helpline (UK/RoI)

- Information Booklets

- Journal: *Reaching Out*

Appendix 2: Support Resources

- Hospital Visits and Support (UK/RoI)

- Discussion Forums

Additional Information
- *Free Telephone Helpline*
  Our Helpline volunteers should be able to address your immediate concerns and answer your questions. You can use the Helpline to organise a local or hospital visit and to order information booklets. See below for the telephone number. From UK, call 0800 374803. From the Republic of Ireland, call 00 44 1529 415278 (normal UK rate applies). Please do not use the Helpline for routine or administrative calls. These should be made on 44 (0) 1529 304615.

- *Information Booklets*
  The Support Group publishes a range of information booklets. While these books are available to read and download at this Web site (see Information pages), you may find the 'printed' word more convenient and it could prove more authorative to medical professionals than a download from the Internet.

- Our Journal *Reaching Out*
  Reaching Out is published three times a year. It is full of news, articles, stories, letters etc. Three free copies are mailed to those who register with the Group. (If you live outside the UK/RoI, you can obtain the journal by airmail by joining the Support Group.)

- *Local Contacts and Hospital Visits*
  The Group has a network of volunteers in the UK

and Ireland who can offer support at a local level. Your local contact will be pleased to organise a hospital visit if that might be considered helpful. A visit by a recovered patient can help morale enormously.

- *Specialist Contacts*
  In addition to its network of local contacts, the Group has contacts who specialise in aspects such as GBS in children, GBS in pregnancy, CIDP, Miller Fisher syndrome, etc. Because of the distances involved, contact will usually be by telephone or e-mail.

- *Mutual Support*
  Use the interactive features of this Web site. You can leave a message in the Guestbook and join the Discussion Forum. Eventually you might consider writing your story or joining the Group and attending our local and national meetings.

- *How to Contact Us*
  All those who contact us will be registered with the Group and will receive three free copies of our journal as well as our literature and other support services. Your details will not be disclosed to others. If you would prefer us not to register your details in our database, please tell us.

  Mail or e-mail. Write to:
  GBS Support Group of the UK, LCC Offices, Eastgate, Sleaford, Lincolnshire, NG34 7EB.
  E-mail: admin@gbs.org.uk.

Appendix 2: Support Resources

The GBS Association of New South Wales, Australia
A non-profit Volunteer Organisation
Registered Charity No. CWD295 Incorporation No. Y13693-18
PO Box 572, EPPING NSW 1710 AUSTRALIA
Phone: 02 9869 1839
Overseas Callers +61 2 9869 1839
Email: guillain@bigpond.com
Website: http://members.ozemail.com.au/~guillain/

The Aims Of The GBS Association Are To:
- increase the awareness of the general public of GBS and CIDP.

- inform medical and rehabilitation staff of the existence of our Association.

- visit and encourage existing and newly diagnosed people with GBS or CIDP.

- maintain telephone support contact numbers for the use of the above.

- distribute literature on GBS and CIDP to patients, relatives, friends and members of the medical profession.

- establish a stock of equipment for loan according to need; and

- raise the necessary funds to achieve our aims.

In our efforts to inform the public about GBS and CIDP, and raise the profile of the Association, information and newsletters are sent at every op-

... A First Step ...

portunity finances allow. Our literature is sent out to General Practitioners, Neurologists, hospital social workers and other health professionals. In addition, attempts have been made to place articles in medical journals. Recently we have produced brightly coloured invitations and posters which we hope to display at hospitals and medical centres.

List of Services
- Extensive Website

- Telephone Support

- Equipment Loan

- Hospital Visitation

- Newsletter: *Recovery*

- Online Reports and Guides

- Information Updates

- International Chapters

Additional Information
- *Example Of Support Available From The GBS Assoc* Initial contact is usually made by a telephone call from a patient, relative, friend or hospital personnel to our Association's Support Secretary.

 Telephone support to the patient, relative or friend who is invariably bewildered by the whole thing at that stage, not knowing what GBS or

Appendix 2: Support Resources

CIDP is or what happens from there on in. Whilst not a doctor, the representative is quite often able to answer any questions that may arise and explain what is happening.

The telephone representative explains what the Association can do regarding hospital visits and support in general. She may redirect them to a person of the same sex, similar age or other particular similarity of symptoms of the patient if they so prefer.

Hospital visits can be arranged through the representative if the patient is in a condition to receive a visit and if they are interested in seeing somebody who has recovered from GBS. Hospital visits continue as long as required and often several Association members may visit over a period of time. We try to match the recovered patient as closely as possible to what we know of the patient currently in hospital.

- *Equipment Loan*
  Equipment loan is available through the Association for any member having difficulties and in need of assistance.

- *Hospital Support*
  Hospital visits can be arranged through Andrea if the patient is in a condition to receive a visit and if they are interested in seeing somebody who has recovered from GBS. Hospital visits continue as long as required and often several Association members may visit over a period of time. We try to match the recovered patient as closely as possible to what we know of the patient currently in hospital.

··· *A First Step* ···

- *Newsletters*
  These are sent out to members 4-6 times per year (level of funds determines frequency). To receive yours, fill out the Membership Form and return to the GBS Association.

- *Reports, Guides, and Information*
  - CIDP — A Short Guide
    This booklet has been written for patients who have been told that they may have CIDP (chronic inflammatory demyelinating polyradiculoneuropathy), and for their relatives and friends. It aims to explain accurately and honestly what CIDP is, and hopefully will answer some of the questions you may have. The degree of severity of CIDP and the way it affects people vary enormously from one person to another. There is no typical CIDP; therefore one general description and one certain prognosis are not possible. This booklet describes the common symptoms.

    - GBS — An Overview for the Layperson
      The Overview is directed to patients with Guillain-Barré syndrome, their families and other interested lay persons. Its aim is to briefly acquaint you with the illness' history, its cause and manner of presentation, describe some of the effects of this disorder on the patient's life and those about him or her.

    - GBS — A GP's Guide to Diagnosis and Management
      This guide is a report on GBS that includes technical information on the condition: definition, aetiolgical factors, pathogenesis, clinical

Appendix 2: Support Resources

features, diagnosis, prognosis, treatment, and management. Also very helpful for the layperson.

- *GBS Association Wish List*
  - More donations and benefactors.

  - More hospital professionals to become members (which would improve their knowledge).

  - Encouraging more people to donate blood and plasma to increase the production of immunoglobulin and getting the need of CIDP patients more recognised and their status raised higher on the priority list.

  - Fewer GBS and CIDP patients.

  - Improved general awareness of GBS and the Association.

  - Last but naturally the ultimate — A CURE FOR GBS AND CIDP.

- *Membership*
  Annual membership of the GBS Association is $16.50 (GST inclusive) for Australian residents and $27.50 (GST inclusive) for Overseas residents. Because of the low membership fee, we look forward to donations of any size. Donations $2.00 and over are tax deductible. Please make all cheques out to The Guillain-Barré Syndrome Association in Australian Dollars and forward to PO Box 572, Epping, NSW, 1710 AUSTRALIA. Members receive a newsletter 4-6 times per year.

IN Group

The Inflammatory Neuropathy Support Group of Victoria Inc.
138b Princess St. Kew, Victoria 3101, Australia
Voice: +61-3-9853-6443
Fax: +61-3-9853-4150
E-mail: ingroup@vicnet.net.au
Website: http://home.vicnet.net.au/~ingroup/

About the IN Group

Supporting sufferers from acute Guillain-Barré Syndrome (GBS) and Chronic Inflammatory Demyelinating Polyneuropathy (CIDP). The IN Group is a non-profit association that provides support to Inflammatory Neuropathy (IN) patients, undertakes research into the cause, treatment and prevention of the illness, and promotes understanding of the condition and its effects.

Our membership comprises current and former patients, relatives, friends and interested members of the public, together with eminent neurologists. We are similar to groups established in New South Wales (The GBS Association of NSW), South Australia (The GBS Support Group Inc. of South Australia), Tasmania (The GBS Support Group of Tasmania), UK (The GBS Support Group of the UK) and the United States (GBS Foundation International).

The IN Group differs from these associations, however, in that we cover both the acute form of inflammatory polyneuropathy — known as the Guillain-Barré Syndrome — and the chronic form — chronic inflammatory demyelinating polyneuropathy.

The Aims of The IN Group
The IN Group is a support group for past and present sufferers of Guillain-Barré Syndrome and CIDP, and aims to spread the message about these rare nerve disorders.

1. To arrange personal visits by former patients to those in hospitals.

2. To provide emotional support to patients and their families.

3. To publish a Newsletter, providing ongoing information.

4. To advise patients regarding resources for vocational, financial and general assistance.

5. To organise group meetings.

6. To encourage research into cause, treatment, prevention and other aspects of the illness.

7. To promote financial support for the Group's activities.

Additional Information
- The IN Group Website has many helpful online newsletter issues and articles.

- The joining fee is $5, and our annual subscription is $10. Members receive a regular newsletter that keeps them up to date on developments.
      Email: ingroup@vicnet.net.au

··· *A First Step* ···

Author Note   Please share this information with other interested parties. If you become a member of any of these groups, mention you learned of them through this appendix. Thank you for your support.

* * *

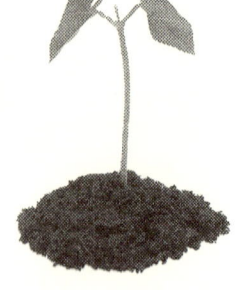

Appendix 3
Internet Information Resources

The following websites have thorough and extensive medical information on GBS discussing the condition, symptoms, diagnosis, possible causes, prognosis, treatment, management, and individual case histories. While much of this infomation is technical, it can be helpful for the layperson to explore.

Thanks again to each of the facilitators, web administrators, and contributors for the use of this information. It is because of you that people with GBS and their families are able to connect globally to conquer this terrible condition. The following information is taken directly from the listed websites and has not been altered except in presentation. Every attempt has been made to ensure the credibility and accuracy of the following information.

GenomeLink: Guillain-Barré Syndrome Hub

Website Address
http://www.genomelink.org/gbs/

... A First Step ...

Description
Extensive list of website links to exhaustive information on GBS from medical communities, associations, organizations, and support groups around the world. Each bullet below is a separate link from the Genome website to the topic or subject listed.

Table of Contents
- Overviews, Full text articles, Diagnosis & Treatment, Research projects, Clinical trials
  - NINDS Guillain-Barré Syndrome Information Page — by the National Institute of Neurological Disorders and Stroke.

  - Guillain-Barré from MEDLINEplus Medical Encyclopedia — updated by Galit Kleiner-Fisman, M.D., FRCP(C), Department of Neurology, University of Toronto, Toronto, Ontario, Canada.

  - Guillain-Barré Syndrome — by Dr. Paul Tinley.

  - Guillain-Barré Syndrome and the 1992-93 & 1993-94 Influenza Vaccines — by Tamar Lasky, PhD, Gina J. Terracciano, DO, Laurence Magder, PhD, Carol Lee Koski, MD, Michael Ballesteros, MS, Denis Nash, MPH, Shelley Clark, MS, Penina Haber, MPH, Paul D. Stolley, MD, Lawrence B. Schonberger, MD, Robert T. Chen, MD.

  - Guillain-Barré Syndrome by David Magnusen

··· Appendix 3: Internet Information Resources ···

- Guillain-Barré Syndrome by the MIT Braintrust Center for Neurological Disorder Information

- Guillain-Barré Syndrome by Loyola University Health System

- Estimated Annual Costs of Campylobacter-Associated Guillain-Barré Syndrome — by Jean C. Buzby, Tanya Roberts, and Ban Mishu Allos.

- Guillain-Barré Syndrome by Charles Miller

- Guillain-Barré Syndrome by Penn State Milton S. Hershey Medical Center

- Guillain-Barré Syndrome by NeurologyChannel

- Guillain-Barré Syndrome by McLeod Health

- Guillain-Barré Syndrome: GBS: Acute Inflammatory Polyneuropathy by The CaF Directory

- Guillain-Barré Syndrome by InteliHealth

- Guillain-Barré Syndrome (GBS) — by Peripheral Neuropathy Program, University of Chiago.

- Guillain Barré Syndrome — linked to vaccination?

- Guillain-Barré Syndrome in Childhood — by Kenneth J Mack, MD, PhD, Senior Associate

Consultant, Department of Neurology, Mayo Clinic of Rochester.

- Guillain-Barré Syndrome by the Guillain-Barré Syndrome Support Group of New Zealand

- Guillain-Barré Syndrome from eMedicine Journal — by David Fanion, MD, Consulting Staff, Department of Emergency Medicine, AO Fox Hospital.

- Intravenous Immunoglobulin is Preferred Therapy for Guillain-Barré Syndrome — by John Frohna, MD., Department of Pediatrics and Communicable Diseases, University of Michigan Health System.

- Childhood Guillain-Barré Study — by John Sladky, M.D.

- Randomized Study of Plasmapheresis or Human Immunoglobulin Infusion in Childhood Guillain-Barré Syndrome — by John T. Sladky, Emory University.

- An Evaluation of the Long-Term Outcome of Children with Guillain-Barré Syndrome — by Darcy Fehlings, M.D., F.R.C.P.(C), and Jiri Vajsar, M.D., Bloorview MacMillan Centre.

- *Directories, Hubs, Web forums*
  - Guillain-Barré Syndrome by DMOZ

  - Guillain-Barré Syndrome by MEDLINEplus

Appendix 3: Internet Information Resources

- Guillain-Barré Syndrome Clinical Resources — by the College of Community Health Sciences, University of Alabama.

- Guillain-Barré Syndrome by YAHOO.

- Guillain Barré Syndrome Web Forum — by the Department of Neurology at Massachusetts General Hospital.

- Guillain Barré Syndrome Foundation Discussion Forums.

- Guillain-Barré Syndrome — by Paulo Andre, MD.

- *Questions and Answers / FAQ*
  - Is there any evidence that Guillian Barré syndrome is associated with ingestion of unpasturized honey? — an answer by Trudy Wassenaar.

  - Is Guillain-Barré syndrome a known side-effect of streptokinase treatment?

  - Guillain-Barré Syndrome by Glaxo Neurological Centre.

- *Case studies and reports*
  - Guillain-Barré Syndrome And The Miller Fisher Variant — by Christopher P. Sobczak, M.D., Safwan Jaradeh, M.D. Medical College of Wisconsin, Milwaukee, WI.

- A 38 year old female presents with complaints of very recent difficulty in walking with weakness of her legs and occasional urinary incontinence.

- *Abstracts*
  - The Swine Flu Vaccine and Guillain-Barré Syndrome: A Case Study in Relative Risk and Specific Causation — by David A. Freedman, Statistics Department, UC Berkeley.

  - Guillain-Barré syndrome: a case report — by John R Pikula, BSc, DC, DACBR, FCCR(C), MSc.

  - Guillain-Barré Syndrome — Diagnosis — by Emory University School of Medicine.

- *PDF, DOC Files*
  - Guillain Barré Syndrome (GBS) — from the Department of Critical Care Nursing, The Ohio State University Medical Center.

  - Guillain-Barré Syndrome: A Mechanistic Study — by Casey Barka.

- *Conferences / Meetings*
  - NIAID Workshop Development of Guillain Barré Syndrome Following Campylobacter Infection — by National Institute of Allergy and Infectious Diseases.

  - Development of Guillain-Barré Syndrome Following Campylobacter Infection — Notes from the Workshop — by Jeff Steinhilber.

- *Support Groups / Associations / Organizations / Foundations*
  - Guillain-Barré Syndrome Support Group UK — their support activities encompass both the United Kingdom and the Republic of Ireland.

  - Guillain-Barré Syndrome Support Group Tidewater Area Virginia Chapter

  - Guillain-Barré Syndrome Foundation International

  - The Guillain-Barré Syndrome Association of New South Wales

  - Guillain-Barré Syndrome Support Group Of NZ

- *Slides*
  - Guillain-Barré Syndrome by Travis Foster

  - Neuromuscular Disorders — by Edward Valenstein.

··· A First Step ···

National Institute of Neurological Disorders and Stroke
NINDS Guillain-Barré Syndrome Information Page

Website
http://www.ninds.nih.gov/health_and_medical/
disorders/gbs.htm

Table of Contents
- What is Guillain-Barré Syndrome?

- Is there any treatment?

- What is the prognosis?

- What research is being done?

- Organizations

- Related NINDS Publications and Information

Washington University Department of Neurology
Neuromuscular: Acute Immune Polyneuropathies

Website
http://www.neuro.wustl.edu/neuromuscular/
antibody/gbs.htm

Table of Contents
- *Classification of Acute Immune Neuropathies*

... Appendix 3: Internet Information Resources ...

- *"Classic" Guillain-Barré Syndrome*
  - Associated disorders
  - Childhood GBS
  - Clinical features
  - Electrodiagnostic features
  - Epidemiology
  - Laboratory features
  - Morbidity
  - Prognosis
  - Prodrome
  - Therapy

- *Other Acute Immune Neuropathies*
  - Autonomic
  - Motor
  - Sensory
  - Miller Fisher Syndrome
  - IgM vs GalNAc-GD1a

- *General topics*
  - Classification: Acute immune neuropathies

- Differential diagnosis: Acute neuromuscular disorders

- General Principles: Acute immune neuropathies

- Treatment of GBS-like syndromes

...

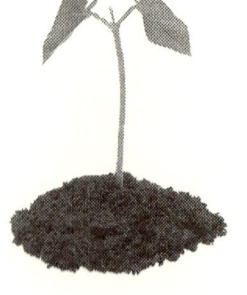

Appendix 4
Reading List

Compiled here is a reading list of books on Guillain-Barré Syndrome. Most of these, like *A First Step*, are autobiographical. I cannot personally recommend them only because I have not read them myself. However, I deemed it important to include them as further resources. This list has been compiled from Amazon.com

Nonfiction / GBS Autobiographies

No Laughing Matter
by Joseph Heller, Speed Vogel
List Price: US $36.80
Paperback: 335 pages
Donald I Fine Publisher
ISBN: 1556114249
(January 1995)

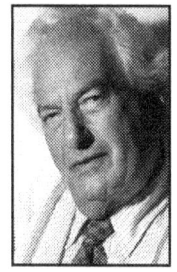

- *From New York Times Book Review:*
  The bestselling author of *Catch-22* teams up with Speed Vogel, his best friend, to describe his battle with and triumph over Guillain-Barré syndrome, a paralyzing disease of the nervous sys-

tem. "Richly amusing... positively cheering."—
The New York Times.

- *Amazon.com Book Description from a Reader:*
No Laughing Matter is a very informative and entertaining piece of writing. Co-authored by Joseph Heller and Speed Vogel (who write alternating chapters) it details the effects of the rare debilitating affliction called Guillain-Barré syndrome. This autobiographical/biographical chronicle passes along a lot of information without once falling into obscure medical dullness.

    Guillain-Barré is a disease that attacks the central nervous system, rendering the victim completely paralyzed. Although what Heller contracted was a mild form of the disorder, in an extreme case mentioned a patient was only able to move their eyes. Recovery is possible from this disease; if it's caught early enough, the patient can be hooked up to a respirator if need be and then slowly rehabilitated. *No Laughing Matter* is two stories. The first is that of Joseph Heller the patient who goes from being in (seemingly) perfect health to being utterly bedridden in a matter of days. The second part of the tale is told by Speed Vogel, a friend of Heller, who took care of virtually all of his financial, legal and personal obligations.

    From reading some other reviews of the book, one might be under the impression that this is a light and fluffy feel-good story of friendship where one will be forced to read numerous passages on the deeper meanings of love and caring. People learning great life lessons by sacrificing much that they have purely in the name of camaraderie. Chicken soup for the soul and novocain for the brain. Fortunately, one couldn't be further from the truth. While the two authors obviously have a great fondness for each other, you won't find any obvious soliloquies on the healing power of friendship. What you will find are people who care a great deal, but aren't afraid to share a lot of good-natured abuse. While in sickness and on the road to recovery, this never feels false or sugarcoated. It's an honest account of what real friendships are made of.

Despite the title, much of the book is laugh out loud funny. Heller may have been bedridden but he didn't lose any of his trademark wit. Celebrity cameos of everyone from Dustin Hoffman to Mario Puzo to Mel Brooks help to liven up an already interesting narrative. Both authors have a warm and engaging style of writing that makes even the more incomprehensible medical jargon understandable. The jokes are great and serve also to counterpoint the feelings of desperation and of loneliness.

The book is extremely intriguing, though there are one or two sections that don't quite work. Heller was going through what appeared to be a fairly messy divorce and the legal proceedings got a little bit complicated. For a section, Heller even reproduces a few pages of the court transcripts in order to show his lawyer in the right. As justified as he may be in including these segments, they aren't nearly as interesting as the rest of the book and pale in comparison.

No Laughing Matter shows us illness from two viewpoints. From Vogel we see the outward appearance of the disease and its effect on Heller. From Heller we experience the sickness firsthand. It's a fascinating dual look at the nature of the affliction. Well worth a read.

No Time for Tears: Transforming Tragedy into Triumph
by Dorris R. Wilcox
List Price: US$24.95
Hardcover: 180 pages
Corinthian Books
ISBN: 1929175078
(March 1, 2000)

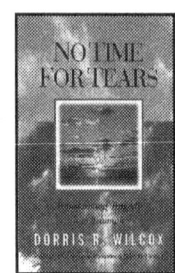

- *Book Description*
  Combining aggressive self-education, massive doses of positive thinking, a barrage of nutritional supplements and unshakable faith in God's healing power, Dorris Wilcox achieved against the odds 95% recovery from Guillain Barré Syndrome, a potentially lethal neurological disorder. She gives sufferers from all debilitating afflictions the tools to acquire and maintain the positive mindset they need to triumph over their own adversity. Also included is an extremely helpful, comprehensive appendix of sources for additional information on Guillain Barr Syndrome.

- *About the Author*
  Born in Dumpling Valley, TN in 1924, and stricken with Guillain Barré Syndrome in 1989, Dorris Wilcox has returned to an active career in interior design and volunteers as a counselor to victims of tragic medical misfortune, including those stricken with Guillain Barré Syndrome. She believes that her faith and a large dose of tenac-

ity pulled her through tough times. A survivor in every sense of the word, she is living proof that if you have a fighting spirit, there is always hope. On November 16, 1990, Dorris received The Patricia Neal Award for Excellence, presented annually to those patients who have resumed an independent lifestyle after recovering from a debilitating illness. She resides in Tennessee.

Nothing But Time
by Judy Light Ayyildiz
List Price: US $21.99
Paperback: 211 pages
Xlibris Corporation;
ISBN: 0738852600
(March 12, 2001)

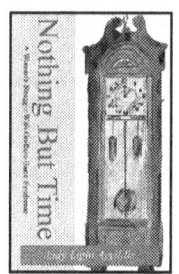

- *Book Description*
  Overnight, everything in her life alters when Judy awakens paralyzed from the waist down by a mysterious illness. As she struggles for the courage to find a way of escape from this well of isolation, pain and powerlessness, her creative imagination takes flight. Armed with insight gleaned from her own stories about events and people in her past and present — told with restrained humor and often with Appalachian flavor — Judy discovers that her spiritual desire to "walk" is stronger than the fear of falling.

- *About the Author*
  Judy Light Ayyildiz was born in Teays Valley, West Virginia in 1941, and graduated from Marshall University with a BA in Music Education. Her husband, Vedii, is a naturalized

US citizen, born and raised in Turkey. For over thirty-five years, they have lived in Roanoke, Virginia, where they raised their children, Kent, Kevin Kamal, and Karen. Vedii continued a private practice in surgery while Judy taught, wrote, acted on stage, engaged in civic work, sang, directed choirs, edited Artemis, and received an MA both in Liberal Arts and in English/Creative Writing from Hollins University.

As a writing consultant during the past twenty years, Judy has created programs in many diverse institutions of learning. She has had honors in poetry, articles, and short stories in literary publications all across the country. Her published work includes three books of poetry and four co-authored supplementary creative writing and critical thinking texts for students and teachers. *Nothing But Time*, Judy's first creative non-fiction work, evolved from a journal that she kept during her plight with Guillain-Barré syndrome in 1985.

Solomon's Porch:
The Story of Ben and Rose
by Jane Riley
List Price: US $19.95
Paperback: 211 pages
AmErica House Book
ISBN: 158851207X
(October 20, 2001)

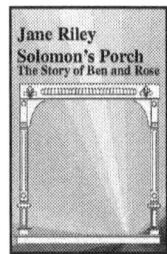

- *Book Description*
  Guillain-Barré syndrome is more than a disease: it is a disaster. *Solomon's Porch, The Story Of Ben And Rose*, is the intimate fictional account of one

family's struggle with an ailment that left Ben Windham paralyzed and his relationships with people changed.

- *About the Author*
  I am a native of south Mississippi, a graduate of the University of Southern Mississippi, and a former teacher in Mississippi public schools. My husband and I taught in Greenville. I am also a graduate of Louisiana Tech University. Currently I reside in north Louisiana with my husband, who has recently retired from teaching music at Tech. We have two dogs and two cats. Our daughter and son-in-law live in south Louisiana. My husband, an ardent fan, said, 'Jane is a well-educated writer who thoroughly researches her subjects. She strives to present realistic situations in her writing.'

Bed Number Ten
by Sue Baier,
Mary Zimmeth Schomaker
List Price: US $32.95
Paperback
CRC Press
ISBN: 0849342708
(May 1989)

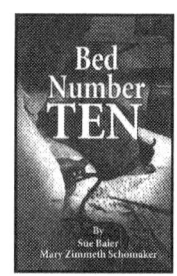

- *Book Description*
  A patient's personal view of long term care. Seen through the eyes of a patient totally paralyzed with Guillain-Barré syndrome, this moving book takes you through the psychological and physical pain of an eleven month hospital

A First Step

stay. *Bed Number Ten* reads like a compelling novel, but is entirely factual.

You will meet:
- The ICU staff who learned to communicate with the paralyzed woman — and those who did not bother.

- The physicians whose visits left her baffled about her own case.

- The staff and physicians who spoke to her and others who did not recognize her presence.

- The nurse who tucked Sue tightly under the covers, unaware that she was soaking with perspiration.

- The nurse who took the time to feed her drop by drop, as she slowly learned how to swallow again.

- The physical therapist who could read her eyes and spurred her on to move again as if the battle were his own.

In these pages, which reveal the caring, the heroism, and the insensitivity sometimes found in the health care fields, you may even meet people you know.

Appendix 4: Reading List

Fiction based on GBS Experience

Masks
by Gloria Hatrick
List Price: US $15.95
Hardcover
Orchard Books;
ISBN: 0531095142
(April 1996)

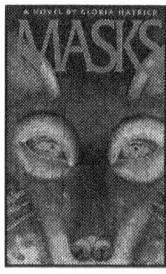

- *From Booklist Book Reviews:*
  Gr. 4-6. When Pete's big brother, Will, becomes paralyzed, Pete communicates with him by using the animal masks their anthropologist father has collected. The masks facilitate an out-of-body experience, with Will becoming the animal represented by the mask. Each encounter becomes more dangerous, however, and Will finds it increasingly difficult to return to his own body. Ultimately, Pete must don a mask himself to save his brother from the brink of death. The point of view jumps rather awkwardly back and forth between the boys, but the idea of two brothers connected by a supernatural bond will intrigue some readers. Pete is a little too perfect; his parents and the other adults in the story are not three-dimensional, but they are presented as responsible and positive characters. Janice del Negro

- *From Kirkus Reviews*
  Summer vacation ends with a tragic turn for the Chisholm family when narrator Pete's older brother, Will, is suddenly and completely par-

alyzed with Guillain-Barré, Syndrome. Both brothers get the runaround: The medical staff talks past them, their parents have low-voiced conversations and try too hard to act normally, and no one will discuss Will's condition in any but general, falsely cheerful, terms. Pete stays loyally at Will's bedside, sure that his brother is aware, and desperate to find some way to help him. Remembering the strange, transformative effects he and his brother had experienced while wearing animal masks from his anthropologist father's large collection, Pete begins sneaking them into the hospital—and they actually elicit small but noticeable responses. Hatrick shifts the narrator's voice to Will to show what's happening; by giving him new ways to visualize movement and to deal with his emotional turmoil, the masks do help; and when a crisis comes, it's the link the masks form with Pete that not only keeps Will alive, but puts him on the road to recovery. The characters here are all stock, but Hatrick's debut, drawn from personal experience, is a stirring, heartfelt tribute to the power of unwavering hope. (Fiction. 10-13)

Nonfiction Reference

Guillain-Barré Syndrome
(Contemporary Neurology Series , No 34)
by Allan H. Ropper, Eelco F.M. Wijdicks,
Bradley Truax
List $72.50
Hardcover
F A Davis Co
ISBN: 0803675720
(February 1991)

- *From Book News, Inc.*
  Clinicians draw on their personal experience and the medical literature to provide a comprehensive view of Guillain-Barré syndrome. The background section covers the history, diagnostic criteria, and epidemiology; other sections cover the neurobiological basis, clinical features, laboratory investigation and differential diagnosis, and treatment and rehabilitation. Especially noteworthy are the details of an approach to managing patients who need respiratory support, which has reduced mortality from 25% to 4% over the past couple decades.

Guillain-Barré Syndrome
(Clinical Medicine and the Nervous System)
by Richard Anthony Cranmer Hughes
Hardcover
Springer Verlag
ISBN: 038719634X
(October 1990)

To Order Additional Copies of *A First Step*

From the Publisher
Trafford Publishing
Suite 6E, 2333 Government St.,
Victoria, B.C., Canada V8T 4P4.
Toll-free: 1-888-232-4444 (Canada & US)
Fax: 250-383-6804
E-mail: sales@trafford.com

Trafford Catalogue #02-0224
Visit www.trafford.com/robots/02-0224.html to order.

Also available at Amazon.com

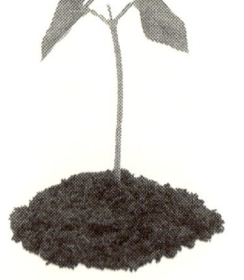

Appendix 5
Guillain & Barré: The Namesakes

In 1916, two French neurologists were serving as doctors in World War I, in the Neurological Centre of the Sixth French Army. Their names were Georges Charles Guillain and Jean-Alexandre Barré. Accompanying them was another doctor whose name was André Strohl.

As they were diagnosing and treating wounded soldiers, they encountered two soldiers who were paralysed. As they tested the fluid levels of the soldier's brains and spinal cords (cerebrospinal fluid), they found their test results and the conditions of these patients differed from test results of other paralysis victims. The two soldiers recovered. The odd situation caused Guillain and Barré to categorize and publish their unique medical findings:

> Concerning a syndrome of the nerve roots with raised levels of protein in the cerebrospinal fluid without cellular reaction. Remarks about the clinical characteristics and graphs of the tendon reflexes.
> —Georges Charles Guillain;
> André Strohl;
> Jean-Alexandre Barré.

Prior to that event, in 1856, another French doctor named Jean Landry discovered a similar type of condition. In 1859, Landry penned the first clear description of the syndrome now attributed to Georges Guillain and Jean-Alexandre Barré. (See earlier reference in Chapter 22, pages 143 and 144).

By 1949 it is noted that most neurolgists generally came to agree that Guillain, Barré and Strohl's description and Landry's were one and the same. The condition is now known as Guillain—Barré Syndrome, perhaps because Guillain, Barré and Strohl formally published their findings. But why Strohl's name was dropped from the formal name is not really known. It seems a shame that both Strohl and Landry are no longer remembered in the name of the disease.

After the War, Guillain became a Professor of Neurology at Saltpêtrière Hospital in Paris, and Barré also became a Professor of Neurology at Strasbourg. Strohl did not pursue neurology, which is, speculatively, perhaps why his name was dropped from GBS. Landry's name, though, still lives on in its own right because of his 'Ascending Paralysis'.

* * *

... Appendix 5: Guillain & Barré; the Namesakes ...

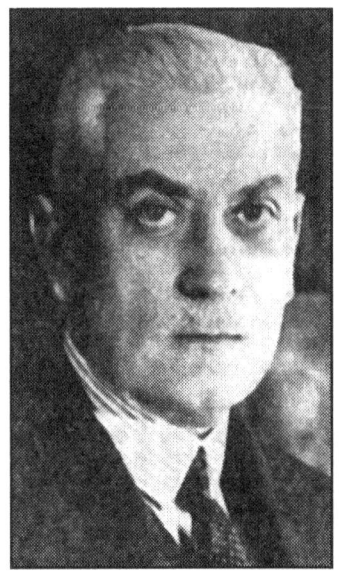

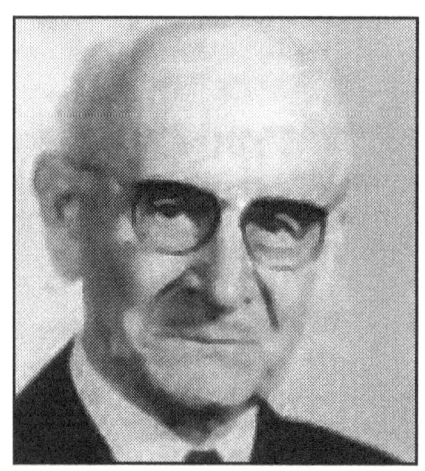

Jean-Alexandre Barré

Georges Charles Guillain.

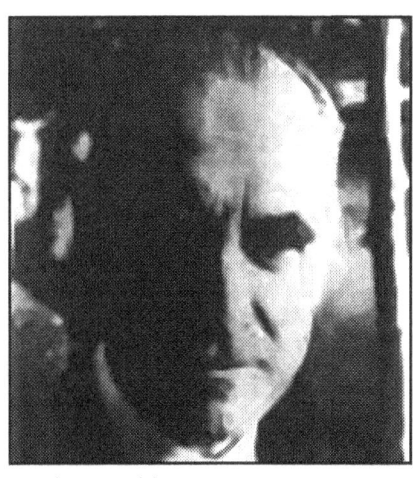

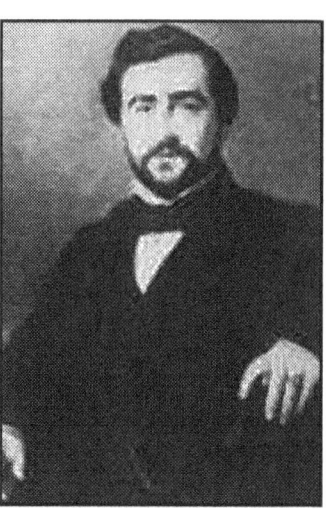

Jean Landry

André Strohl

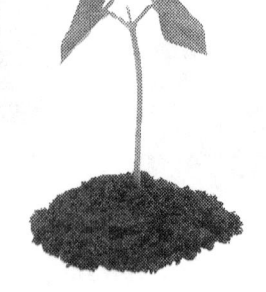

Appendix 6
The Index

Note: Page numbers followed by letter '*n*' refer to endnotes.

A
Acute chronic axonal GBS, 18, 102
Acute dysimmune polyneuropathy, 11
Acute idiopathic polyneuritis, 11
Acute idiopathic polyradiculoneuritis, 11
Acute inflammatory polyneuropathy, 11
Alphabet boards, in communication systems, 44
Anger, 120 – 121
Arm rack, 77
Autoimmune system, 16 – 17
Autonomic nervous system, 13
Axon, 12, 13
Axonal GBS, 13, 37, 102
Ayyildiz, Judy Light, 369 – 370

B
Baier, Sue, 371 – 372
Balance, 333*n*
Barré, Jean-Alexandre, 10 – 11, 143, 379 – 380
Bed Number Ten (Baier), 371 – 372
Beds
    and bedsore prevention, 124, 135, 145

transfer between wheelchair and, 23 – 24, 27 – 28, 38, 105, 118, 135, 160, 332n
Bedsores, 124, 145
Benson, Robert and Estelle, 337
Birthday celebration, 30
Bladder stones, surgery for, 31
Brain, function in GBS, 13, 177
Brain damage, 128
Bronchoalveolar lavage, 22
Burk, Kopel, 47 – 49, 57 – 58, 329n, 330n

C

Call button, 123, 124
Campylobacter jejuni/coli, as cause of GBS, 15, 16
Cancer diagnosis scare, 31
Card system of communication, 47 – 48
Catheter, 51, 83, 330n
Cerebrospinal fluid, in GBS diagnosis, 10 – 11
China, GBS variants in, 13, 16
Christmas holidays, 95 – 96, 98 – 99, 331n
Chronic axonal GBS, 102
Clothing, 62, 64
Communication, 330n
   alphabet boards, 44
   Burk, Kopel on, 47 – 49
   card system of, 47 – 48
   computers and, 165
   early in paralysis, 21 – 22
   talking aids, 69 – 79
Communication and Altered Perceptions (Burk), 47 – 49, 57 – 58
Communication journal, 53
Computers, for communication, 165
Control, desire for, 91, 139, 157
Cot transfer, 105, 118, 332n
Coughing, 130

Cytomegalovirus, as cause of GBS, 15

D
Dentures, 76, 77, 109, 119 – 120
Diabetes, 104, 125, 129
Discomfort sensations, 133
Disorientation, 23, 62
Dreams, 24, 177 – 317
Drinking, 77 – 79, 82

E
Electrical currents, in physical therapy, 44
Elevator, in home, 149 – 150
EMG tests, 29, 35, 140
England, trip to, 2 – 3
Entertainment, 41
Epstein-Barr virus, as cause of GBS, 15
Europe, trip to, 1 – 5
Exercises
   rehabilitative, 166
   strengthening, 168
   stretching, 124
Eyebrow movement, as communication system, 21 – 22

F
Falling, 166
Family conferences, 24, 29, 49 – 50, 90 – 91, 145, 331*n*
Fear, 49, 123, 169, 329*n* – 330*n*
Feeding tube
   change from nose to stomach, 32 – 33
   removal of, 120
Feedings
   intravenous, 23, 32 – 33

liquids, 77 – 79, 82
solid foods, 120, 139, 160
Finland, GBS outbreaks in, 16
Fitness
    exercising, 124, 166, 168
    level of, 69
    and recovery from GBS, 18
Flu vaccines, as cause of GBS, 15, 18
Foothills Hospital, 6
    intensive care unit of, 21 – 24
    nurses in, 23
    rehabilitation program of, 104, 121, 123
    transfer from, 27
Friendship, 324
Future, planning for, 41

G
The GBS Association of New South Wales, Australia, 343 – 347
GenomeLink: Guillain-Barré Syndrome Hub, 353 – 359
Goals, importance of, 321 – 322
Guillain, Georges, 10 – 11, 143, 379 – 380
Guillain-Barré syndrome (GBS)
    acute chronic axonal, 102
    alternative names of, 11, 143
    axonal, 13, 18, 37, 102
    causes of, 15 – 18
    characteristics of, 9
    defining, 12 – 13
    diagnosis of, 6 – 7, 37
    differences from brain damage, 128
    differences from quadriplegia or spinal cord injury, 127 – 128
    first sign of, 5 – 6
    historical background of, 9 – 11
    Miller-Fisher variant of, 143
    nerves affected by, 11, 12 – 13

nontransmissibility of, 17
severe acute chronic axonal, 18
variants of, 13, 143
Guillain-Barré Syndrome (Clinical Medicine and the
  Nervous System), 375
Guillain-Barré Syndrome (Contemporary Neurology
  Series, No 34), 375
Guillain-Barré Syndrome Foundation International, 337 – 339
Guillain-Barré Syndrome Support Group UK/RoI, 339 – 342

H
Hallucinations, 24, 177 – 317
Hand splints, 125
Handi-bus, 333n – 334n
Hatrick, Gloria, 373 – 374
Hawaii, trip to, 109
Health insurance, 128
Heller, Joseph, 365 – 368
Home
  alterations to, 141, 149 – 150
  assessment of, 129
  early visits, 134 – 135, 140 – 141
  first visit, 133 – 134
  overnight visits, 144 – 145
  return to, 157 – 162
Home caregivers, 334n

I
Illness, before onset of GBS, 2 – 5, 17
Immune system, strength of, and severity of GBS, 18
Immuno-gamma globulin, 22, 24, 28
IN Group, 348 – 349
Infection precautions, 49
Injections, as cause of GBS, 15

Insect stings, as cause of GBS, 15
Insulin, 22
Intensive care unit
    dreams in, 177 – 178
    at Foothills Hospital, 21 – 24
    reflections on life in, 87 – 89
    at Rockyview General Hospital, 27
    transfer from, 110, 113 – 114, 117 – 118
Internet resources, 353 – 362
Intravenous feedings, 23, 32 – 33
Itching, 123

J
Job loss, 78
Jordan, GBS outbreaks in, 16

L
Landry, Jean B.O., 10, 11, 143 – 144, 379 – 380
Landry's ascending paralysis, 11, 143 – 144, 380
Lip-reading, 43, 50, 90
Liquids, reintroduction of, 77 – 79, 82

M
Masks (Hatrick), 373 – 374
Medications, 22, 28, 76, 85, 91, 129
Miller-Fisher variant of GBS, 143
Molecular mimicry, 16 – 17
Morphine, 22, 28
Mucus plug, 83
Mycoplasma pneumoniae, as cause of GBS, 15
Myelin, 12, 13, 17

N

National Institute of Neurological Disorders and Stroke (NINDS), web site of, 360
Neck brace, 28, 30, 279
Nerves
   affected by GBS, 11, 12 – 13
   coming back, 123, 128, 133, 140, 141
   regrowth rate of, 35
New Year's, 100
No Laughing Matter (Heller & Vogel), 365 – 368
No Time for Tears: Transforming Tragedy Into Triumph (Wilcox), 368 – 369
Nothing But Time (Ayyildiz), 369 – 370
Nottingham Forest, 64, 81
Nurse staffing issues, 49, 50, 124, 128, 334n
Nurse-to-patient ratio, 124
Nursing shift changes, 87
Nursing staff, gaining attention of, 177

O

OB sling, 137
Occupational therapy, 23, 129, 137, 138, 154, 167
Oxygen saturation, 106
Oxygen therapy, 119, 129 – 130, 331n. *See also* Ventilator

P

Pain, as sign of recovery, 71, 74, 133
Palma de Mallorca, Spain, 4
Panic attack, 72, 78
Paralysis
   onset of, 21
   pattern of recovery from, 22
Peripheral nerves, 12
Pessimism, 169

Pet therapy, 89
Physiotherapy, 23, 44, 137, 138, 153 – 154, 167
Planning for future, 41
Pneumonia, 2, 22, 90, 289, 292
Porphyria, as cause of GBS, 15
Porta de Pollenca, Spain, 4
Positive attitude, 37, 118
Priddis Greens Golf and Country Club, 1, 30, 324
Protein, in cerebrospinal fluid, in GBS diagnosis, 10 – 11
Pulse oximeter, 106

Q
Quadriplegics, 127

R
Reaching Out, 341
Recovery
    expectations for, 118
    length of, 35
Reflexes, 6, 10
Rehabilitation, 104, 137 – 139
    end of, 167 – 170
    start of, 77 – 79
Rehabilitation program, at Foothills Hospital, 104, 121, 123
Rehabilitation table, 77, 97, 105
Resource shortages, 128
Retirement, 78
Riley, Jane, 370 – 371
Rockyview General Hospital, 6
    nurses in, 23
    transfer from, 121
    transfer to, 27

S

Sense of humour, 21 – 22, 51, 54, 57 – 58, 88, 137 – 138, 177
Sensory nerves, 12 – 13
Severe acute chronic axonal GBS, 18
Signs, definition of, 10
Sitting up, 51, 75
Sneezing, 130
Solid foods, reintroduction of, 120, 139, 160
Solomon's Porch: The Story of Ben and Rose (Riley), 370 – 371
Spain, trip to, 3 – 4
Speech therapy, 50, 61 – 62, 71
 and tracheotomy valve device, 69 – 79
Spinal cord, function in GBS, 13
Spinal cord injury, 127
Springtime, 137
Staffing issues, 49, 50, 124, 128, 334n
Stair climbing, 167, 168
Standing, 82 – 83, 118, 135, 333n
Staphylococcus aureus, 22
Steinberg, Joel S., 9 – 13, 15, 17, 329n
Stretching exercises, 124
Strohl, Andre, 10 – 11, 379 – 380
Strychnine, in GBS treatment, 11
Surgery, as cause of GBS, 15
Swallowing test, 82
Swine flu vaccine, as cause of GBS, 15
Symptoms, definition of, 9
Syndrome, definition of, 9 – 10

T

Television, 41
Tick bites, as cause of GBS, 18
Tilt table, 77, 97, 105
Trach cork, 84, 97, 101, 102, 103, 104, 110, 330n – 331n
Trach cradle, 89, 91, 97, 101, 331n

Tracheotomy, 23
   healing of site, 158
   leaking of, 33, 34
   removal of, 130
   valve for speech in, 69 – 79
Transfer, between bed and wheelchair, 23 – 24, 27 – 28, 38, 105, 118, 135, 160, 332n
Transfer board, 135, 138
Travel
   as cause of GBS, 18
   to Europe, 1 – 5
Trip, first outside hospital, 95 – 96

U

University of Calgary Health and Fitness Program for the Handicapped, 168
Urinary tract infection, 71

V

Vaccines, as cause of GBS, 15, 18
Ventilator, 28, 31, 32
   air leaks in, 83
   alarm of, 330n, 335n
   weaning from, 41 – 43, 73, 74, 105, 106, 110, 113, 332n
View from hospital window, 88, 177
Viral infections, as cause of GBS, 15
Vitamin C, 90, 97
Vogel, Speed, 365 – 368
Voice-activated software, 165

W

Walking, 153 – 154, 168 – 169

Washington University Department of Neurology, web site of, 360 – 362
Weight loss, 59
Wheelchair
   adjustment to, 27 – 28
   electric, 134, 158, 159, 321
   home accessibility, 141, 149 – 150
   increasing time spent in, 33
   new model, 38, 105, 106, 124
   transfer between bed and, 23 – 24, 27 – 28, 38, 105, 118, 135, 160, 332*n*
Wheelchair tolerance, 139
White blood cell count, 22, 63
Wilcox, Dorris R., 368 – 369
Winer, J.B., 10 – 11, 143 – 144, 329*n*, 333*n*

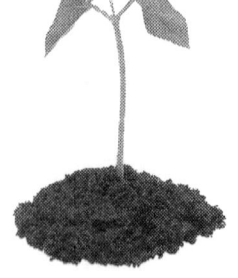

Appendix 7
About the Author

* * *

Brian was born in Derbyshire, England in 1928. He was educated at the West Bridgford Grammar School, Nottingham. After two years of service in the British Army, he embarked on an accounting career, which eventually led to a senior financial position in Salisbury, Wiltshire. In 1977, having achieved his career ambition, he emigrated for the second time, to the 'Blue Sky country' — Alberta, Canada — with his wife and three daughters, seeking new challenges.

It was in June 1998 when he met with the catastrophic life-threatening illness, Guillain-Barré Syndrome. At the time of his frightening encounter with that disease, Brian was a healthy 'young' sixty-nine year old International Sales Manager. He was an enthusiastic golfer, even if, in his own words, not particularly good. In addition, he enjoyed various other hobbies, each one calling in its own way for physical fitness. These included gardening, model railroading, and walking. He had, and still has, a keen interest in nature. He loved to spend much of his leisure time walking and enjoying the wildlife that was so abundant in the area close to his home in Calgary.

His book, *A First Step — Understanding Guillain-Barré Syndrome*, is a personal account of a battle for survival against an acute, chronic form of that rare disease, and his subsequent determination to return to as normal a life as possible. His story should be an inspiration to others.

Brian S. Langton first hit upon the idea of writing a book while lying, virtually paralysed, in a rehabilitation ward. He had earlier been stricken with a particularly serious form of Guillain-Barré Syndrome, sometimes referred to as G.B.S., and had already spent over seven months in intensive care, more than six of those months on a ventilator for breathing assistance. He had recovered his ability to speak, and was becoming used to entertaining visitors by recounting some of the dream sequences he had experienced during his period of hospitalisation. He was interested and encouraged by the positive messages he appeared to be providing to his visitors.

Many of the dreams were quite hilarious, in spite of Brian's serious predicament, and it occurred to him that a collection of them would make for interesting reading. It had also become evident that few had experience of G.B.S., and he was constantly being made aware of just how rare the illness was, and of the nursing community's appetite for knowledge about the Syndrome. It was this realisation which prompted Brian to seriously consider writing a book, not just about the dream sequences but to produce a sort of handbook on G.B.S., suitable for medical professionals, caregivers, G.B.S. patients and relatives, alike.

Upon eventual discharge from hospital, Brian carried these thoughts home. He could not write at that time. It was only just possible for him to move his right arm in a limited way from the shoulder. His recreational therapist had arranged a one finger splint to allow him to use a computer keyboard by pressing one key at a time, but it would take more than that to write a book, or so he thought. It was not until a student caregiver convinced him that he was physically capable of writing the book he was contemplating, even if it meant using 'voice software' and possibly, if the worst came to the worst, by the one finger typing method.

Thus encouraged, and in spite of no writing experience, Brian, with the help and encouragement of that student, commenced work on his book at the start of the new millennium, January 2000.

● ● ●

www.ingramcontent.com/pod-product-compliance
Lightning Source LLC
Chambersburg PA
CBHW020721180526
45163CB00001B/58